ALSO BY DAN KENNEDY

The Wired City: Reimagining Journalism and Civic Life in the Post-Newspaper Age (2013)

The Return of the Moguls: How Jeff Bezos and John Henry Are Remaking Newspapers for the Twenty-First Century (2018)

With Ellen Clegg:
What Works in Community News: Media Startups, News Deserts, and the Future of the Fourth Estate. (2024)

More information at www.dankennedy.net

Critical Praise for *Little People*

"*Little People* … is extraordinary, a heartfelt yet not maudlin story of the achondroplasia — dwarfism — of Mr. Kennedy's young daughter."

— *The Wall Street Journal*

"Part family memoir and part cultural inquiry, the book traces perceptions of dwarfism throughout history, shedding light on our society's convoluted reaction to difference. *Little People* is brutally honest and intellectually riveting. Kennedy's writing shifts seamlessly from humor to heartbreak, and he's not afraid to disturb his readers."

— *Child Magazine*

"Dan Kennedy writes in a friendly, trustworthy voice about difficult topics: difference, prejudice, and disability. *Little People* has the form of memoir and the effect of social commentary. Its power is cumulative. Using his own parental anxiety and curiosity as a bridge, Kennedy makes unfamiliar experience accessible."

— Peter Kramer, best-selling author of *Listening to Prozac* and *Spectacular Happiness*

"Kennedy's an ideal guide. . . . He takes us on a journey that is both singular and universal for any parent of a child who is 'different.'"

— *The Boston Globe*

"So much for us to consider as we go through this extraordinary book — how fate and chance determine the circumstances of our lives — all told in wonderfully affecting and summoning language by a thoughtful and introspectively energetic father and writer who shares with us a family's life and in so doing helps us to become his companions in human understanding."

— Robert Coles, best-selling author of *The Moral Intelligence of Children* and the Pulitzer Prize-winning *Children of Crisis*

"Dan Kennedy's writing is clear, measured, and generous, and reflects both the seriousness of his intellectual enterprise and the profundity of his love for his daughter. This book is about the processes of acceptance, and tells how one learns to tolerate difference, and then to cherish it."

— Andrew Solomon, best-selling author of *The Noonday Demon* and winner of the National Book Award

"Had *Little People* . . . existed when my daughter was born it would have saved me months of research and hours of soul searching."

— *Salon*

"Kennedy's deeply rooted hope for Becky's meaningful place in this unpredictable world drives him to seek answers to 'what it means to be different — the good, the bad, the myths, the truths.'"

— *The Providence Journal*

"Kennedy's book is reminiscent of Michael Bérubé's powerful memoir and reflection on his experiences as a father of a child with Down syndrome, *Life As We Know It.* He mixes together his personal story with an examination of the social, ethical and philosophical issues raised by dwarfism. This combination works well because it deepens the significance of his own experience, and makes the abstract issues more accessible."

— *Metapsychology Online*

"Kennedy, a journalist by trade, leaves few aspects of being a little person unexplored — from circus history and the fate of a Jewish dwarf in Nazi Germany to the current-day exploitation of little people in porn films and the annual convention of the Little People of America."

— *Publishers Weekly*

LITTLE PEOPLE

Learning to See the World Through My Daughter's Eyes

DAN KENNEDY

Photographs, reviews, essays, and additional features:

www.littlepeoplethebook.com

Original hardcover edition published by Rodale in 2003

Paperback ISBN: 978-0-578-47445-8

For my parents,

the original Dan and Barbara Kennedy,

who died much too young.

They would have loved their grandchildren.

And their grandchildren would have loved them.

CONTENTS

Foreword

By Becky Kennedy

For as long as I can remember, I have been different from everyone else. The reason is that I have achondroplasia. Even though that is the most common form of dwarfism, I am still different from most people, since dwarfism itself is very rare. Achondroplasia affects somewhere between one in 15,000 and one in 40,000 people. When I was growing up, and even now as an adult, I have been noticed because of my dwarfism. Some people — mostly little kids — stare at me and whisper things such as "Look at her!" and "Why is she so little?"

When I was a kid, the comments and the stares bothered me a lot. But after years of experiencing it, and knowing that it's mostly from children, I've gotten used to it. I really don't mind at all. In fact, by the time I became a teenager, I realized that when little kids make comments, it is my duty to educate them and explain to them the reason why I am so short, especially since they have probably never seen a dwarf before.

Because I rarely get to meet other people with dwarfism in my everyday life, I feel blessed to be part of an organization like Little People of America, which sponsors regional and national conferences as well as camping trips and other activities. I fit right in with everyone because they know what I'm going through. I have friends who are dwarfs, and, like me, they have experienced curious kids staring at them and making comments. So I feel like that's even more reason to educate people about dwarfism. Also, whenever I am at an LPA event, I can just be myself and not worry about having to explain to people why I'm short. Regionals and camping trips are a time for having fun and relaxing, not answering questions.

My life as a dwarf hasn't just affected me emotionally and mentally, but also physically. Like probably every other dwarf in the world, I sometimes have trouble reaching items that are above my head. Sometimes I need help; sometimes I can get it myself if I have a stepstool available. But occasionally even that's not enough. For instance, the cabinets in our house are so high that, whenever I want to make dinner, I need a stepstool and a pair of tongs to grab things that are on the upper shelves. Sometimes the best solution is simply to move items I need regularly to a lower shelf.

Like most young adults who are around my age, I want to be independent, so I try to do things by myself. There are times, though, when it's easier said than done. I mean, I appreciate a little help every once in a while, but it is frustrating to have to rely on others as often as I do. But I am proud of myself because even though I need help more often than I'd like, I usually find a way to get it done. To me, there's always a way. It's just a matter of figuring out what the right way is.

At twenty-six, dwarfism doesn't seem to affect me as much as it did when I was a kid. I guess I've just gotten used to finding out how to do things a little differently from most people, along with asking others for help. That was especially true in learning how to drive. It took me a while to get my license, mostly because my dad and I had to share his car until I got my own. That was a challenge because, every time I wanted to drive, we had to attach pedal-extenders and make adjustments to the driver's seat so that I would more or less feel comfortable. It was frustrating because it took about ten minutes just to get the pedal-extenders on. Since my dad and I were sharing his car, this routine had to be repeated every time I wanted to drive.

It wasn't until I got my college graduation present from my parents — a car — that I was finally able to be as independent as I wanted to be. We visited a few dealers until we finally found a car that felt like it was practically made for me. The pedal-extenders fit like a glove, I felt comfortable in it, and the best part of all was that I never have to make adjustments because I'm the only person driving it. I thanked my parents multiple times, and, for weeks, I thought to myself, "I'm looking at my car with my own eyes, and I still can't believe it."

Dwarfism has also affected my attempts to find a job. I've applied, and even had some interviews, but unfortunately was turned down quite a few times. Getting a first job can be difficult for anyone, but I think it's especially hard for dwarfs. I say that because, since we are of short stature, there is only so much we can do on our own without the help of a stepstool or other adaptations — and too many employers don't want to take a chance on someone who has to do things differently. Fortunately, I was recently offered a job at a supermarket not far from where we live. My family couldn't have been more excited or thrilled for me.

Back in the early 2000s, when I found out that my dad was going to write a book about dwarfism and about me, I was excited and honored, as any fifth-grade girl probably would be. That changed after the book came out and I was asked to be interviewed at school by a television news station. I was very nervous, especially after I found out that they wanted to follow me around during school hours. I felt different enough from my classmates, and the last thing I wanted was a pair of reporters coming to my classroom and worrying about how my classmates would react. Fortunately, the reporters were understanding and agreed to interview me after school hours, but while I was still in the classroom, doing schoolwork.

As an adult, I still feel honored that my dad has written this book. After reading it for the first time in years, I also feel elated and blessed just to be alive after learning about the medical problems I struggled with during the first three years of my life, none of which I remember. It also kind of scared me. My health is good today, and I can't imagine the hard times we went through.

My dad's book also makes me feel proud of both myself and my dad. This book means the world to me because it teaches people of all sizes what it means to be a dwarf and how, in a way, dwarfs are just like everyone else — only shorter.

Introduction to the Third Edition

On a rainy day in May 2018, Rebecca Elizabeth Kennedy graduated from Bridgewater State University in Southeastern Massachusetts. It had been a long road. Several years earlier she had earned an associate's degree from Landmark College in Putney, Vermont, which helps students overcome their learning disabilities. In Becky's case, her learning issues may be related to her dwarfism. She was twenty-five by the time she walked up to the podium at Bridgewater — not especially old for a newly minted college graduate, but older than many of her peers. She was ready, finally, to begin the next phase of her life.

In the course of writing *Little People* more than fifteen years ago, a theme I returned to repeatedly was our hopes and expectations that Becky would be able to lead a normal, fulfilling life. She has. After graduating, she moved back home with us (not permanently, she insists). She drives a car outfitted with pedal-extenders. She is getting involved in our church and meeting new people. She is diligently looking for work. And though she knows she faces discrimination from prospective employers who assume she will not be able to meet the physical requirements of whatever job she is applying for, she keeps at it. In fact, she received an offer just recently, something she and we are pretty excited about.

For the purposes of this book, perhaps the most important change in this, the third edition, is that her own voice is now being heard. I asked her to write the Foreword, and she has done what I think you'll agree is a wonderful job of expressing what it has been like to grow up with dwarfism, the challenges that come with it, and what it's like to have your father write a book about you. I am thrilled to be able to offer her perspective. Her degree from Bridgewater is in English, and she aspires to write for a living. She is off to a good start.

Our lives are very different compared to the early 1990s, from which much of the emotional energy of this book derives. Back then, Becky was fighting for her life as she struggled to overcome breathing problems, a consequence of her having been born with achondroplasia, the most common form of dwarfism. By the time she was three years old, though, she was fully recovered and has enjoyed good health ever since. She is four feet tall, with exceedingly short arms and legs, and she sways from side to side as she walks. Yet her dwarfism, though hardly an inconsequential part of her life, does not define her.

If our lives have changed over the past few decades, so, too, has the way dwarfism is depicted in popular culture. When Becky was a baby, there was the occasional magazine or television success story about a little person making his or her way in the world. More frequently, though, were stories about Hank the Angry, Drunken Dwarf, a sidekick of Howard Stern's who has since died. Or midget wrestling. Or midget porn.

Those negative portrayals have all but disappeared. A few years ago you couldn't flip through the cable channels without coming across TLC's upbeat series of reality shows on people with dwarfism

— *Little People, Big World*, starring Matt and Amy Roloff, whom I have known for years, and who were interviewed for this book; *Little Chocolatiers*; and my personal favorite, *The Little Couple*, whose co-star, Jennifer Arnold, was a pediatrician who was profiled in one of the first magazine stories I read about dwarfism after Becky was born. Peter Dinklage, an actor with dwarfism who has starred in movies such as *The Station Agent* and in HBO's fantasy series *Game of Thrones*, has emerged as a far more positive representative of the dwarf community than poor Hank.

And yet the forces of reaction are real. *Little People* is not a political book. But after eight years of the Obama presidency, a time when we began to take it for granted that an African-American president was in the White House and when tremendous strides were made in areas such as same-sex marriage and transgender equality, it is impossible not to observe that we are now dealing with a very different reality. President Donald Trump has denounced in hateful terms Muslims, immigrants, and anyone who dares to oppose him. He mocked a disabled journalist while a crowd of supporters hooted in delight. In 2018 he even appointed a judge to the D.C. Circuit Court of Appeals who had written several times in support of the humiliating and dangerous practice of dwarf-tossing, arguing that it was a matter of personal choice — never mind that it puts the person tossed at risk of serious injury and holds an entire class of people up to ridicule. For people with disabilities and other differences, this is truly, as Dickens put it, the best of times and the worst of times.

From its inception, this book had two intended audiences: families affected by dwarfism and other disabilities, whom I hoped could learn from our experiences; and a wider readership that might be interested in the history, culture, and science of a rare and little-understood condition.

My original publisher, Rodale, allowed *Little People* to go out of print a number of years ago. The second edition, which I made available through print-on-demand technology, was released in 2010. This third edition is virtually unchanged except for this Introduction and Becky's Foreword. Additional content is available at www.littlepeoplethebook.com, where you can find photographs, reviews of and feature stories about the book, and essays about dwarfism that I have written over the years.

Difference creates community, and by far the most rewarding aspect to having a child with dwarfism has been becoming part of the dwarf community — as interesting and engaging a group of people as I have known. We would not have chosen dwarfism for our daughter. Yet we are grateful for the friendships she has made through Little People of America, the leading organization for people with dwarfism and their families. *Little People* is not just our story, but theirs as well.

Dan Kennedy
West Medford, Massachusetts
March 2019

Chapter One

An Unexpected Journey

From almost the moment we were told that our beautiful new daughter was a dwarf, I've been on something of a quest — a quest to find meaning and purpose in Becky's having a life-altering genetic difference. I don't want to suggest that I've been looking for meaning in her *life*. That's a given. I've always believed that she has the same potential, the same opportunities, the same chance to succeed or fail, to be happy or sad, as anyone else. But I wanted more. I wanted to know *why* she was different — or, to be more accurate, why her *particular* difference was so much more obvious than those that affect most of us. And I wanted the answer to that question to be positive, uplifting, life-affirming.

Maybe it's a function of fatherhood, of the ever-so-slight distancing from family life that is imposed on men by biology and social conditioning. For my wife, Barbara, who's more focused on Becky's immediate needs, such questions of meaning are a waste of time and energy. *She is who she is.* But for me, forever part participant, part observer, the search for meaning is central.

My compass is the idea of diversity, of the belief that human variation is in and of itself a positive good, and that, though dwarfism will surely cause Becky problems, there are beneficial aspects to it as well. Greater empathy. Strength of character. Even service to humanity: she could be carrying genes whose purpose is unclear at the moment but that someday might prove beneficial. But is that really an honest way of looking at Becky's dwarfism? Or am I just kidding myself, rationalizing, trying to create a comforting fantasy out of a complicated reality?

By now you'd think I would know better. After all, Becky is my only daughter, someone I've looked at, admired, and worried over every day of her life. You'd think it wouldn't require the puzzled reaction of strangers, of the outside world, of a culture that simultaneously celebrates and fears diversity, to pull me out of my reverie and force me to focus on the facts of the matter: That at the age of ten she is no taller than an average five-year-old. That her head is already much bigger than her older brother's, with a heavy, prominent forehead. That her arms and legs are impossibly short, that her butt sticks out, and that she sways back and forth, waddling, when she walks. That she is a *dwarf* not a poster child for some abstract ideal of diversity.

Not that I ever lose sight of this, exactly. In some ways, the realities of Becky's dwarfism are always with me. Every day I think about the dwarfism-related breathing complications that nearly killed her when she was a baby and that held sway over her first three years. And I know that dwarfism continues to alter her life in ways both large and small — from the slight hearing loss that makes it difficult for her to learn, to the miniature clarinet that she plays because she can't reach the bottom keys on a standard-size instrument. But these are side effects, consequences of her dwarfism, not dwarfism itself. To strangers, she is — as a physician's article on dwarfism that I once read so charmingly put it — a *funny-looking kid.* To us, though, her dwarfism has little to do with how she looks and everything to do with the ways it has changed — not diminished — her life, and ours.

Her learning disability makes it hard for her to understand what she reads, but she is brimming with empathy for others. Her tastes in television shows, movies, and computer games lean toward those of a much younger child, yet she has such a sense of responsibility that she will do her chores and her homework without having to be told. Her size often relegates her to playing with kids half her age, yet she is so outgoing with adults that she thinks nothing of picking up the phone and pitching Girl Scout cookies to friends of ours whom she's only met a few times. These are tangible signs of who she is, of a personality and an identity shaped partly by her dwarfism, mostly because no two kids are alike. The labeling — the idea that she is a dwarf, and that's all she is; that her individuality is subservient to how differently she happens to be put together — well, that's what I often lose sight of. Except on those occasions when others remind me.

On Labor Day weekend in 2002, right after Becky's tenth birthday, I took her to her favorite amusement park, a place in New Hampshire called Story Land, near Mount Washington. It was a rare father-daughter day; my son, Tim, had gone camping with friends; Barbara stayed home. As with the TV shows and movies that Becky watches, Story Land is geared mainly for children several years younger than she. But the reason she likes Story Land more than, say, Six Flags is strictly practical: she is just tall enough to be allowed on every ride.

I resolved to pay attention on this cool, sunny Sunday — to stand aside as much as I could and take in the scene. What I saw was a revelation — not that I should have been surprised. People were staring. There was a little pointing — not much — and some long, incredulous looks. Shuffling through the slow-moving lines for the more popular rides, I noticed people looking at Becky, whispering, wondering.

As I was waiting to order lunch, a woman came up to me and asked how old Becky was. Now, I've gotten those questions before, and normally I suggest that the person ask Becky herself. Many adult dwarfs say there's a common assumption that because they're short, they must be mentally disabled as well. To counter that, I like to nudge people into engaging with Becky, to experience her outgoing personality and her wit. This time, though, Becky had found a couple of kids to play with, and they were running in and out of a mock jail with rubber bars, shouting and laughing. So I told the woman that Becky was ten, and waited for the look of confusion, followed by enlightenment, that invariably follows. She then asked me the politically correct term for — well, *you* know. I should have replied "Becky," but my tongue ran ahead of my brain. "'Dwarf' is fine," I said. She seemed satisfied and walked away.

Later I thought, *What an odd encounter.* Not unpleasant, mind you. The woman had been friendly and inquisitive, and there was nothing about her demeanor to suggest that she thought Becky was to be pitied or looked down upon. Still, her boldness in coming up to a perfect stranger and asking why his daughter was — well, a *funny-looking kid* — communicated the unspoken message that Becky is public property, and that her parents are obliged to explain her to the world. And I realized that obligation would eventually have to be taken on by Becky herself.

I've heard dwarf adults say that, from childhood on, they've been treated as if they're always on display, never anonymous, never able to blend into the crowd. I once heard a woman — an attractive thirty-nine-old mother of four who happens to be four-foot-two — lament that she can't even get out of the mall without fielding questions about what it's like to be a dwarf.

Whenever Becky and I go about our business near our home in Danvers, a suburb on Boston's North Shore, people — kids and adults alike — are always stopping, rolling down their car windows, waving, and saying, "Hi, Becky!" Because of her hearing problems, compounded by a certain congenital obliviousness, I sometimes have to give her a nudge before she'll wave back. And at least half the time she can't tell me the names of the people who've just greeted her. They know her; she doesn't know them. They're anonymous; she's not. They can choose whether to wave or not, to say hello or not, to drive on by or not. But she's expected to be polite and friendly at all times, to acknowledge the presence of others because they have chosen to acknowledge hers.

I have come to understand that Becky must learn to be an ambassador — a visiting dignitary from the Land of Dwarfism, always upbeat, always polite, always *on.* It may not be fair. It may not even be possible. But it's there, all the time, tied up in our cultural fascination with difference, with otherness. Dwarfism, in effect, functions as a metaphor for that fascination, inspiring laughter, fear, revulsion, condescension — but never the sort of half-conscious non-reaction we normally experience when encountering ordinary people going about their ordinary lives. Dwarfs, too, are ordinary people leading, for the most part, ordinary lives. Yet they invariably provoke an extraordinary reaction.

This book tells Becky's story. But it also tells my story, a father's story — and that of a people, a *race* even, whose members are no different from anyone else except for the way they look, and yet whose difference has cast them in the role of perpetual outsiders. Above all, it is the story of my quest to find meaning in that difference.

Rebecca Elizabeth Kennedy was born on August 29, 1992. My education about dwarfism — and about our culture's conflicted attitudes toward people who are visibly different — began a week and a half later, in a nondescript office in downtown Boston. I can't say there was any real sense of drama in that moment. Barbara and I had already been told that Becky had achondroplasia, which is the most common form of dwarfism. We knew there was little likelihood of that diagnosis being wrong. Still, when the pediatrician had suggested we take Becky to see a geneticist, we readily agreed, figuring we'd learn — well, who knows?

Maybe somewhere in the backs of our minds — or, to be more honest, in the back of *my* mind — I held out the possibility that there really was nothing wrong with Becky. That the doctors who had examined her in the local community hospital couldn't tell the difference between normal and abnormal. Becky was a fairly typical-looking newborn, and at that point I found it impossible to imagine — emotionally, if not intellectually — that her genetic programming would stop her from growing when she reached the four-foot mark. How, I wondered, could they be so sure?

That last sliver of psychic defiance evaporated as soon as we were called into the geneticist's office. The doctor — a well-manicured, middle-aged woman in a business suit, not a white coat or stethoscope in sight — put us at ease with her direct, friendly manner. She explained that x-rays of the bones in Becky's arms and legs had confirmed her achondroplasia. She examined Becky and showed us several subtle characteristics that proved she had achondroplasia: a slight separation between the third and fourth fingers of each hand — sort of a permanent Mr. Spock greeting — and fatty deposits on the small of her back. There were less subtle signs, too, such as the soft spot on the top of her head, which wasn't really a spot at all but rather encompassed pretty much her entire skull from the ears up.

There was more. Following this brief examination, we reconvened in the geneticist's office, whereupon her voice took on a portentous tone.

"I want you to know," she told us, looking grave, "that there really wasn't anything you could have done about this."

A slight pause ensued before I responded, "What do you mean?"

She explained that achondroplasia couldn't have been detected by amniocentesis or any other tests given early in pregnancy to determine whether the fetus has some sort of genetic disorder. (This is no longer true, but, for now at least, it might as well be: even though the genetic mutations that cause achondroplasia and several other forms of dwarfism have been discovered in recent years, they are not yet included in routine genetic screening — as, say, Down syndrome is for women who are in their mid-thirties or older.)

For a moment, I was dumbfounded in the literal sense of that word, at a loss as to what she was driving at. Then, one of us — I'm no longer sure whether it was Barbara or me — figured it out, and asked her if she meant there was no way we could have found out in time to terminate the pregnancy. I'm pretty sure that's how we put it, too — "terminate the pregnancy." There was, after all, a living, breathing baby in the room, wiggling in Barbara's arms, and we were talking about her. Somehow it would have seemed obscene to say "abortion" out loud, even though Becky was many months away from understanding that or any other word.

"Uh, yes," the geneticist responded, looking distinctly uncomfortable. Given the choice, she added, many expectant parents — maybe most — would choose to terminate. Well, *we* wouldn't, we replied with some defiance.

And with that, our appointment began to draw to a close. The doctor recovered enough of her composure to congratulate us on having such a beautiful baby — no small thing for parents who've just been told their child has a major genetic condition — and gave us some literature from Little People of America, an organization about which we would learn much in the months and years to come. She also told us that, in all likelihood, Becky would enjoy normal health, normal intelligence, and a normal life span. As we were leaving, Barbara and I admired Becky anew, and asked ourselves, with a mixture of smugness and incredulity, how could anyone talk about terminating *this*?

But is it really so simple? Our convictions, after all, couldn't be separated from the healthy baby who was with us right at that moment. What about months earlier — say, during the first trimester of pregnancy, when, at least according to legal and cultural norms, the stakes were lower? What if we had learned Becky would be born not with dwarfism but, rather, a fatal genetic defect, or one of those horrible degenerative conditions that seem to crop up regularly on the front page of the local paper, with photos of a sick-looking kid and his stoical parents beneath headlines such as "Benefit Walk Scheduled for Courageous Youngster"? What if it were something more difficult and challenging and heartbreaking than mere short stature — like mental retardation or blindness or deafness or some profound disfigurement that would frighten children, disturb adults, and require years of chancy surgery?

For that matter, what if we had known that within five months of being born, Becky would nearly die when a common virus invaded her respiratory system, overwhelming airways that, because of her dwarfism, were smaller than a normal baby's and twisted in such a way that her oxygen supply was nearly cut off. That she would have to undergo a tracheostomy and spend two difficult years breathing through a tube in her throat. That our home would be transformed into a miniature medical center, filled with air tanks and oximeters and beeping alarms and nurses who watched Becky at night so that Barbara and I, exhausted from tending to her needs during the day, could get something like a normal night's sleep. What would we have said if we'd known all this when Barbara was ten weeks pregnant?

I'm framing this as though the issue were abortion, but it isn't. Rather, this is about a considerably more profound issue: the differences between human beings, whether we fear those differences, whether we value them, whether we would stamp them out if given the opportunity. The geneticist had brought up another matter as well. She told us there was an experimental operation, pioneered in Russia, to lengthen a dwarf's arms and legs so much that they appeared almost normal. (I'm using the word "normal" advisedly; I would later learn that those in the dwarf community prefer to use the term "average size" to describe folks who are not dwarfs. As with race, gender, and sexual orientation, there is a whole vocabulary of politically correct language preferred by many dwarfs and their families that is violated at one's peril.) The surgery, she explained, was extremely painful and sometimes resulted in life-threatening side effects such as infections and nerve damage. She was — to her credit — adamantly opposed to putting a child's life at risk simply to make her appear more like everyone else. Yet she added that she had had parents in her office requesting, demanding information about the surgery, insisting that their child needed longer arms and legs in order to enjoy a normal — that word again — life.

Now, the case against such surgery isn't airtight. Dwarfs must move about in a human-made world designed for people between five feet and six feet tall. If you're four feet tall, you get stared at. But it goes well beyond that. You also can't reach ATMs (not all of them, anyway), drive a car without special adapters, adjust a showerhead, or get the cereal off the top shelf without a step stool. A dwarf's short arms make personal hygiene difficult as well. Some dwarfs who've undergone limb-lengthening surgery are quite happy with the results, and they say that reports of pain and infections have been exaggerated. But limb-lengthening is, at root, a statement of deep cultural discomfort with difference. It's sadly ironic that it is most successful when performed on adolescents, who desperately want to look like their peers. By the time a dwarf is in her twenties, limb-lengthening is much more difficult. Of course, by then, her maturity and self-image may well have developed to the point that she'd no longer want the surgery in the first place.

We live in a culture of entitlement, and one of those supposed entitlements is the right to have perfect children — that is, children who are conventionally attractive, intelligent, even-tempered, and well-behaved. We all expect our children to be like those who populate Garrison Keillor's Lake Wobegon, where everyone is above average. With adults embracing the ethic that bigger breasts or thinner thighs or a longer penis are just a surgeon's scalpel away, it's not surprising that they would transfer these attitudes to their offspring as well. Some kids with Down syndrome undergo surgery to make their eyes look less "mongoloid," and studies show that a substantial minority of people — perhaps 10 percent or so — would choose abortion if they learned that their fetus would have a genetic predisposition to obesity. *Obesity!*

These attitudes are juxtaposed against a backdrop of incredible scientific change. The decoding of the human genome will eventually make it possible to diagnose in utero all sorts of conditions and predispositions and characteristics. Within a few years, or a few decades, it may be possible to screen routinely for, say, the hundred most common genetic conditions, a category that would include achondroplasia and several other types of dwarfism. Will it become just as routine for doctors to recommend termination? What if insurance companies withdraw coverage from would-be parents who refuse to abort a fetus with a genetic condition?

What happens a few decades or a few centuries from now, when we are well past the primitive abort-or-don't-abort conundrum and instead routinely alter the genes of embryos to eliminate a predisposition for stupidity or fatness or manic depression or homosexuality or a mean streak or a tendency to watch holographic sitcoms while talking to your friends on the videophone instead of doing your homework *right now*, young lady? Will we all be the same? Will we all be above average?

There are thought to be somewhere between thirty thousand and fifty thousand people in the United States with some type of dwarfism, of which there are about two hundred or more different varieties. The definition of dwarfism itself is difficult to pin down. Little People of America defines it as a medical or genetic condition that usually results in an adult height of four-foot-ten or less, with no distinction made between men and women. Medical definitions vary. I saw one that attempted to define dwarfism in statistical terms: someone whose height is in the lowest 0.25 percent of the general population. By this measure of dwarfism, the adult height limit for men would be five feet and one-half inches, and for women, four feet eight inches.

But if you go to a Little People of America gathering, you'll quickly see that there's no need to pull out a tape measure: the vast majority of dwarfs in LPA are about four feet tall, with a substantial minority who are quite a bit shorter than that. In part, this may be because people who are close to the limit — taller dwarfs, if you will — see no need for LPA. Mainly, though, it's because the most common types of dwarfism result in an adult height of somewhere between three feet and a little more than four feet tall.

By far the most common type of dwarfism is achondroplasia, responsible for perhaps two-thirds or more of all cases. Studies show that about one in every twenty-six thousand to forty thousand babies is born with achondroplasia. The vast majority of the parents — around 85 percent — are not themselves dwarfs; that is, they are "average size."

Because achondroplasia is a genetic condition — a genetic defect, really, though some in the dwarf community don't like such harsh terminology — it is present at the moment of conception. It makes no sense for me to wish Becky didn't have achondroplasia because without it, she wouldn't be Becky. An achondroplasia-free child would have required a different sperm (the mutation is believed to originate with the father) or a different egg, and thus a person with a completely different genetic endowment. Some damaged bit of genetic material was present at the creation during our lovemaking, and unlike most such occurrences — which are incompatible with life, and which result in miscarriages, many of them so early that the woman doesn't even realize it's happened — this one did not prevent a fetus from taking hold in the womb.

Until the genetic basis for achondroplasia was discovered, it was thought that it somehow involved a failure of the cartilage to develop into normal bone. In fact, the word *achondroplasia*, which is derived from Greek, means "without cartilage formation." Now scientists understand that achondroplasia is actually caused by a gene mutation that affects the body's ability to regulate how much bones should grow and when they should stop growing.

Achondroplasia belongs to a broader group of dwarfing conditions known as skeletal dysplasias, all of which are genetic disorders that affect bone development. There is essentially no treatment; giving growth-hormone shots does little or no good, although such shots can help with a rare condition known as growthhormonedeficient (GHD) dwarfism, which is caused by a hormonal imbalance rather than a bone disorder. (GHD dwarfs, whose proportions are the same as an average-size person's, used to be called "midgets," though that is now regarded as an offensive term. "Dwarf" and "little person" are generally acceptable in describing a person with any type of dwarfism.)

The genetic mutation that causes achondroplasia is dominant, a term you may remember from high-school biology classes about Gregor Mendel and peas. Each of our inherited characteristics comprises two genes, one from our mother and one from our father. When a characteristic is dominant, only one of the two genes needs to be affected. An average-size person cannot be a carrier of achondroplasia, since if you inherit just one mutated gene, you're a dwarf. Thus, average-size parents who give birth to an achondroplastic child might as well have gotten a personal visit from Ed McMahon bearing a check with a dollar sign followed by lots of zeroes: it is the result of a random genetic mutation, and has nothing to do with their own family history. (As far as Barbara and I know, there have been no dwarfs in either of our families.)

Many other genetic conditions, including some types of dwarfism, are recessive, meaning that you have to inherit mutated genes from *both* parents in order to have the condition; if you inherit just one mutated gene, you are unaffected, though you are, indeed, a carrier. Conceive a child with another carrier and that child has a one-in-four chance of inheriting the genetic mutation from both parents, and, therefore, of having the condition.

When someone with achondroplasia has a child with a person who is average-size or who has a different type of dwarfism, the likelihood of passing on achondroplasia increases to 50 percent. In fact, such mixed couples are just as likely to have a healthy achondroplastic child as are couples in which *both* partners have achondroplasia. That is because of an immutable fact of genetics known as double dominance.

Here's how it works. The child of two achondroplastic parents has a 25 percent chance of not inheriting the mutation from either parent, and would thus be average-size (an unaffected gene from each parent); a 50 percent chance of being a dwarf (an affected gene from one parent, and an unaffected gene from the other); and a 25 percent chance of inheriting the mutation from both parents, the aforementioned double-dominant condition, which inevitably leads to death shortly after birth.

Such heartbreaks could not be prevented until 1994, when a research team led by the late John Wasmuth, of the University of California at Irvine, identified the genetic mutation that causes achondroplasia. Concerned that his discovery might be misused, he invited officers of Little People of America to the news conference at which he announced his findings, and expressed the hope that prenatal testing for achondroplasia would only be used by dwarf couples seeking to learn whether their child would inherit the fatal double-dominant condition. Still, Wasmuth clearly knew his discovery would eventually make it more difficult for achondroplastic children to come into the world. As that geneticist in Boston had told us in 1992, two years before Wasmuth's announcement, *There really wasn't anything you could have done.* But that was then. When Barbara was pregnant with Becky, we opted not to have her undergo amniocentesis. But if accurate prenatal screening that was not potentially harmful to the fetus had been offered, and if such screening included achondroplasia — well, as I said earlier, who knows? I'm reasonably sure we wouldn't have been congratulated and given literature about Little People of America; instead, I imagine, we would have been pressured, subtly or otherwise, to choose abortion. All under the additional pressure of knowing that with each passing week our decision would become that much more difficult.

In those first months after Becky was born, I'd often find myself walking around with my right hand extended in front of me, level, palm down, squinting, measuring, adjusting. I was commuting by train and subway that fall, so I saw hundreds of people every morning. I'd look for the short ones, the women in particular, and try to figure out their height, where the tops of their heads would be if they were standing right next to me, how that compared with the unexpected new reality of our lives. I'd squint again, move my hand up, then down. *Here? Maybe a little lower? Look at that woman over there. She couldn't be much more than four feet. She doesn't look too bad. We could live with that.*

Later, when my focus had shifted from the train station to the hospital, from *How tall will she be?* to *Will she come out of this okay?*, I understood that I'd had it all wrong. I'd been holding my hand out in front of my chest; I should have moved it down to my waist. The short women I'd been looking at were just that — short — and nothing more. They weren't burdened by anatomical anomalies that could cause life-threatening medical problems, complications that could develop over a period of years or, as we were to learn, at a moment's notice. They didn't get stared at (except by me), pointed to, called "Midget!" behind their backs — or right to their faces. They didn't need to ask for help in pressing an elevator button. They didn't drag themselves up the curb as though they were working out on a singularly diabolical exercise machine.

In other words, they weren't *dwarfs*. Becky, I realized, was the first dwarf I'd ever seen, not counting television or maybe once or twice in the flesh, in a crowd, off in the distance, somewhere, maybe. As an adult, Becky would be four feet tall, give or take a couple of inches — and yes, her head would be larger than most people's, and yes, her arms and legs would be tiny, and yes, she'd waddle when she walked.

We could live with that. I mean, what choice did we have?

I've long since put my hand back in my pocket. Height is not an issue in our home. When I was growing up, my father would measure me every so often, his pencil marks clearly visible on the doorjamb next to the bathroom for years after I'd reached my full six-foot height. Not so in our house, not even for Tim, who's well on his way to being a six-footer himself. From the time she was old enough to understand, we've been telling Becky that size doesn't matter, that she would grow up just like everyone else, even though she wasn't going to grow *up*. She struggled with this, told us she didn't want to be a "dorf" because she didn't want to be a kid forever. She kept this up even though she'd seen dwarf adults, even though one friend, in particular, had been to our house on several occasions with her own adopted son, who's also a dwarf, and had gone out of her way to show our daughter the pedal extensions she uses so that she can reach the gas and the brake in her car — the ability to drive, of course, being sure proof of adulthood.

Having worked so hard to convince Becky that height didn't

matter, it would have been hypocritical or even harmful for us to cluck approvingly over each quarter-inch she'd managed to gain, to mark it on the wall as if it were some sort of accomplishment. The motto of Little People of America is "Think Big." It's a harmless, benign message from the organization's early days in the late 1950s and early 1960s, an artifact of a less contentious, less politically charged era. But I suspect if LPA members today were to take a second look at their motto, they'd come up with something different.

Len Sawisch, a psychologist and disability-rights activist from Michigan who's also a dwarf, says that telling dwarfs to "think big" makes about as much sense as telling African-Americans to "think white." Think big? Hey, short is beautiful, baby.

Chapter Two

Life Saving

Barbara and I met as students at Northeastern University, fell in love, and got married in our early twenties — then waited ten years before having kids. Partly this was a matter of circumstance: I wanted to put off having a family until I had gotten my master's in American history at Boston University, a five-year slog through night school. Then my parents became terminally ill, first my father, followed by my mother; and I, as an only child, spent most of my nonworking time taking care of them. After my mother's death — too soon, really, even to begin to process all that had happened — I started a quarterly magazine in Boston's northern and northwestern suburbs, an ill-conceived venture that flopped in less than a year. That was followed by a year of personal struggle: unemployment, deep depression, and gradual recovery.

Barbara and I have always had something of an odd-couple relationship: I am loud and talk too much; she is quiet, and there are times when she hardly talks at all. I run and hike; she'd rather go to the mall. I like Bob Dylan and Bruce Springsteen; she prefers Simon & Garfunkel and George Winston. What we share — what we've shared almost from the time we met — is a fierce devotion to each other, a devotion that's all the stronger because it's hard to explain. She got me through this dark period, picking me up at a temporary job I had and driving us to the beach with bag lunches, slowly, gradually, pulling me through it. Some marriages can fall apart during such times; ours grew stronger.

When we were finally ready to start a family, we discovered that there's a lot more to getting pregnant than just having sex — and that staying pregnant is even harder. After a year of trying, Barbara finally became pregnant, only to suffer a miscarriage sometime during the winter of 1989-90, an event I am ashamed to say that, because of my own preoccupations, I barely remember with anything other than a vague feeling of relief.

By the spring of 1990, though, she was expecting again, and this time we were both ready. Timothy Daniel Kennedy was born on January 15, 1991. He was so strong, and his birth so uneventful, that a nurse actually suggested in the delivery room that Barbara get dressed and go home. Two weeks later, I began work as a copy editor at the *Boston Phoenix*, a venerable alternative weekly newspaper. The angst of the previous year had given way overnight to the American dream: a good job and a brand-new baby.

Timmy's health was remarkable, and I can honestly say that I never saw it as something we were entitled to. For most of the 1980s, I had worked as a reporter for the *Daily Times Chronicle*, in Woburn, Massachusetts, and covered a landmark federal trial over the dumping of toxic waste, a case made famous in Jonathan Harr's 1995 book, *A Civil Action.* During those years I became friends with Anne Anderson, whose insistence on finding out why her son Jimmy had gotten leukemia — and why he'd died — was the driving force behind the lawsuit. Anne was and is a friendly and kind woman, but her sadness was never far from the surface. My experience in Woburn taught me never to take any child's health for granted. I marveled at Timmy's strength and looked at it as a gift. He breezed through check-ups. He was walking by one, running not long after that, a loud, curious presence, disdaining naps for fear that he would miss something, scampering around the kitchen table and laughing while Barbara and I ate our supper.

Barbara had always wanted three kids; I, having grown up without brothers or sisters, was a bit skeptical, but I certainly wanted two. Barbara came from a big family: she had two brothers and a sister, and they and her parents — along with spouses and grandchildren — all lived within a few blocks of each other in Colonie, New York, a suburb of Albany. Barbara was the only member of her extended family who'd moved away — who'd escaped, we liked to joke. At Tanski family gatherings, it was Barbara who was loud and boisterous, and I who was quiet and withdrawn. Big families were alien to me. Yet I had some vague regrets at not having a brother or sister to talk to, especially with my parents gone. I figured we'd go for two and then decide later on a third. Barbara figured that having a third child was something that would take care of itself.

"I could have twins," she would tell me, laughing. "My father was a twin."

"Well, that would be okay," I replied.

"Or we could have two — and *then* I could have twins."

"Jesus . . ."

One fact was indisputable: we couldn't have child number three (or four) until we'd had number two. And having waited as long as we had for Timmy, we knew we were running out of time. Less than a year after Timmy's birth, we were expecting again; but that pregnancy, too, ended in miscarriage. By now we were in our mid-thirties, with conception and pregnancy becoming more difficult with each passing year. With the help of Clomid, a fertility drug, and daily temperature monitoring, by early 1992 Barbara was pregnant once more. We hoped for the best and set our sights on August, the due date.

Yet even though we didn't know at the time precisely what was going on, there were signs throughout that something was not quite right. Barbara's pregnancy with Timmy had been almost entirely without complications, but with Becky it was one thing after another. Because of Barbara's two miscarriages, her obstetrician put her on progesterone, which Barbara had to administer to herself in the form of vaginal suppositories. Next, it was discovered that she had placenta previa — that is, the placenta was partially blocking the cervix, a situation that could result in dangerous bleeding and that would require a Cesarean section. Fortunately, and surprisingly, the placenta moved on its own accord, and no C-section was necessary.

In the final weeks, Barbara grew absolutely huge. With Timmy, her size had stayed well within normal range, but with Becky she swelled with amniotic fluid — characteristic, we were later told, of a genetic bone condition, although at the time her obstetrician seemed unconcerned. That expanse, in turn, gave Becky so much room to swim that she never really moved into position for delivery. Thus, Barbara had to be induced with Pitocin, a synthetic version of oxytocin, the hormone that causes contractions. Barbara got contractions, all right — violent, nauseating contractions that doubled her over while she walked up and down the hospital corridor with an IV drip in her arm.

Becky's dwarfism was actually detected before she was born, though no one realized it. A routine ultrasound showed that Becky's arms and legs were shorter than expected — or, as the radiologist put it, her head and torso appeared to be at thirty-six weeks, whereas her arms and legs were at twenty-eight weeks. He chalked up the anomaly to getting a "bad angle" because of the excess amniotic fluid, which made it difficult for him to move Becky into position for an accurate picture. We accepted that explanation; at least, I have no memory of having any serious doubts.

Becky was born at Beverly Hospital late on a Saturday afternoon. She had inhaled meconium — fetal poop — during delivery and had to be rushed to the special-care nursery lest she come down with pneumonia. She was a beautiful baby, eight pounds, two ounces, nineteen and a half inches long — just a half-inch shy of her brother's length at birth. Certainly, at least at first, there was no suspicion that there was anything wrong other than the meconium in her airways and a touch of hypoglycemia.

I went home for a few hours to check on Timmy, who had been staying with neighbors. By the time I returned, everything had changed. A doctor from Boston, filling in at the special-care nursery for the weekend, was concerned about the size of Becky's head. It was, she said, clearly larger than normal. It could be brain damage; it could be dwarfism. We were horrified by the prospect that our brand-new little girl might have something seriously wrong with her, and — no doubt as a self-defense mechanism — I have completely forgotten the chain of events that led to brain damage being ruled out. I just remember being profoundly grateful that the worst that could happen didn't happen. Which left the possibility of dwarfism, a notion as exotic and strange to us as if we'd been told she was from another planet.

Timmy had been a perfect-looking newborn; his birth was so easy that he didn't even have the misshapen head common with justdelivered babies. Barbara and I both knew that Becky, though reasonably normal-looking, was — well, off a bit. It was hard to tell whether her arms and legs were shorter than they should be, but there was no doubt that she had an unusual head: large and flat, with a triangular appearance when you looked down at the top. That evening, I picked up Timmy from the neighbors' and, after putting him to bed, anxiously called Barbara's obstetrician and told him of the concerns that had been raised. He doubted the possibility of dwarfism, but my feeling of relief did not extend much past the moment when we ended our conversation and I hung up the phone.

Achondroplasia in a newborn is subtle, and in some cases it can take weeks or even months before suspicions are raised and a diagnosis is made. If it hadn't been for that one doctor in the nursery, I think I would have believed — willed myself to believe — that Becky was fine. I suspect Barbara would have asked more questions. To this day she recalls sitting with Becky in the nursery just seven hours after she'd been born and wondering about her slightly off-kilter appearance. "I remember holding her that night and *knowing* there was something wrong," she says. Still, it could have been quite a while before we got the right answers. Dwarfism is not, after all, the sort of thing a local hospital runs into every day.

What is normal? More specifically, what is a genetic difference and what is a genetic defect — and how do you distinguish between the two? Does it matter? In a word, yes. In language and in the real-life attitudes that language reflects, differences are good, defects are bad; differences are to be nurtured, defects eliminated. To eliminate a defect that causes real suffering is obviously an unalloyed good. But if one person's defect is another person's difference, then the moral calculation changes considerably. And if the defect/difference can't be eliminated without also eliminating the person, well, that's another order of magnitude altogether.

Some of these judgments are easy to make. Consider eye color. Brown is dominant and blue is recessive, meaning there are more people with brown eyes than blue. I'm oversimplifying, and I'm not even mentioning those whose eyes are green or gray or utterly unique, but indulge me. If brown eyes are the default mode for the human race, are people with blue eyes somehow defective? Of course not. Blue eyes work exactly the same as brown ones. Mine happen to be blue. Of far more significance, though, are the facts that I've had to wear glasses since I was nine, that middle age forces me to switch back and forth between two pairs when I'm reading, and that an allergy often makes my eyes dry and itchy and uncomfortable. Eye color? Who cares?

Or take race. Through some combination of genetic attributes, people of European, African, and Asian ancestry all look quite different — from the pigmentation of their skin to the shapes of their noses and eyes to the color and texture of their hair. But despite the efforts of some to pretend otherwise, we know that racial differences are morally and intellectually neutral, meaningless — and of little importance when compared to other aspects of our genetic make-up. Scientists say that the genetic differences between Europeans and Africans, for instance, are less pronounced than the differences among various African ethnic groups. Obviously the genetic differences that are the most visible are not necessarily those that are the most profound, or that help determine who an individual *is*.

Now turn the needle over to the other end of the dial. Down syndrome, quite clearly, is a genetic defect — a condition created by an extra chromosome that causes mental retardation and myriad other problems, such as heart abnormalities, hearing deficiencies, and short stature. (Some reference books actually refer to Down's as a type of dwarfism. That's not necessarily wrong, but it seems beside the point.) People with Down's often enjoy good, meaningful lives, especially when brought up in a loving home environment rather than the institutions they were typically warehoused in several generations ago. Still, no reasonable person would call Down syndrome a mere genetic difference on the order of eye color or ethnicity.

The same is true of genetic defects that do not manifest themselves until adulthood, such as those responsible for Huntington's chorea (the disease that killed Woody Guthrie), amyotrophic lateral sclerosis (affecting Lou Gehrig, the physicist Stephen Hawking, and Morrie Schwartz, of *Tuesdays with Morrie* renown), and certain types of breast cancer. No one would call these mere genetic differences. And even though you could construct an argument that Gehrig, Schwartz, and Hawking have had a more significant and lasting legacy than they would if they'd never gotten ALS, it is nevertheless true that their genetic defect had an enormous, and damaging, effect on their lives.

Finally, turn the needle back to the middle. This is the part of the dial occupied by dwarfism. Difference or defect? Diversity or pathology? It is a politically charged debate with consequences not just for the dwarf population, but — in an age of prenatal testing and the promise (and threat) of genetic engineering, at a time when our increasing *acceptance* of difference is matched only by our growing ability to *eradicate* it — for all of us.

Nowhere does this debate rage louder than within the dwarf community itself. On the Dwarfism List, an Internet forum with nearly eighteen hundred subscribers that I had a hand in founding and continue to help run, there is little agreement on the difference/defect divide. Some frankly define dwarfism as a genetic defect. Others are quick to respond, "God doesn't make mistakes." This is supposedly the show-stopper for the religiousminded, though it conveniently circumvents the matter of whether, say, infants born without brains are evidence that God occasionally takes a day off.

The whole reason for the debate, I suspect, is that although dwarfism is a disability (in itself a controversial assertion in some circles), it's a different *kind* of disability. In contrast to a person who is blind, or deaf, or uses a wheelchair to get around, a person with dwarfism — in most instances, anyway — is fully in possession of all of her physical abilities. A dwarf looks not so much like a person with a disability as she does a member of a different race, or even a different type of human. As the medical anthropologist Joan Ablon writes:

> Within the context of populations labeled as physically different, the situation of the dwarf is made more complex and ambiguous for the average-sized perceiver than is that of a person with a missing limb or an impaired sensory organ, since in the

> case of many dwarfs, there is nothing really "wrong" or dysfunctional about any one part of them. The person is just smaller, or in the case of disproportionate dwarfs, the body is in a different form, but it is all there, and all *part of a piece*, with each part fitting into a harmonic, although different, whole.

Thus, according to Ablon, dwarfism is a disability, but it's a *socially constructed* disability. People with dwarfism are disabled not by the lack of some physical function, but by a culture that perceives there is something wrong with them — "something wrong, but not *too* wrong," Ablon writes — and that discriminates against them by denying them opportunities that it routinely grants to the average-size majority. Such discrimination can take the form of refusing to alter the human-made environment — lowering door handles, elevator buttons, toilet seats — in order to accommodate dwarfs' short stature. Or it can be more explicit: refusing them a job or admission to a school, or staring and pointing and laughing at them in public places.

But wait. Most disabilities, not just dwarfism, are socially constructed to a greater or lesser degree. It seems intuitively correct to say that a dwarf is not disabled in the same way that a blind person is disabled, but is that really true? For instance, if an ATM is so high that a little person can't reach it, how is that any different from a blind person's being unable to see it? If a deaf person attends a lecture and cannot hear, then he is disabled; but if there is a sign-language interpreter standing next to the speaker, then his disability disappears — or becomes meaningless, which is more or less the same thing. For some years now, a segment of the deaf community has denied that deafness is a disability of any kind. Activists have sought to elevate American Sign Language to the level of, say, English or French, and have denounced cochlear implants — surgically inserted devices that restore hearing in certain types of deafness — as the cultural equivalent of genocide. Personally, I think a middle position is appropriate. Deafness, like blindness or paralysis, is a real, physical limitation. But thinking about it primarily within its social context — a context that the hearing majority has the power to change — helps us create a better, more inclusive world.

Dwarfs, too, have real physical limitations. They aren't just short. They aren't just disproportionate. They don't just walk differently. They are disabled, in objective fact as well as cultural theory. The most dramatic example is that the opening inside a dwarf's spinal column is barely big enough to accommodate the spinal cord. In some cases — particularly with advancing age, but sometimes in young children — "barely big enough" gives way to "too small," and the only way of preventing paralysis or even death is to saw the spinal column open and remove chunks of vertebrae. Dwarf adults sometimes suffer through years of tingling and weakness and pain, trying to put off surgery as long as possible; it certainly isn't the sort of thing anyone would want to go through twice, though some do. And there's more, much more. Dwarfs can't extend their arms fully at the elbow. Children tend to get bowed legs, which can make walking difficult and painful, and which has to be corrected by surgery. Some dwarfs, especially kids, have hydrocephalus, "water on the brain." In most cases it's mild enough to warrant nothing more than monitoring and measuring. But in a few rare instances, the condition is severe enough that a shunt has to be surgically inserted, draining excess fluid from the skull cavity to the abdomen. And — as we were about to learn with Becky — sometimes, again mainly with kids, the airways are so small that they can get easily overwhelmed by a common respiratory virus, turning what should be no more than a bad cold into a life-or-death struggle.

Keep in mind that I'm talking only about achondroplasia. As I observed earlier, at least two-thirds of all dwarfs are "achons," as they are sometimes called. But something like two hundred different types of dwarfism have been identified, some of them unnamed and specific to one individual, some quite disabling. People with the most common types of dwarfism other than achondroplasia — diastrophic dysplasia, pseudoachondroplasia (despite its name, not genetically related to achondroplasia at all), and spondyloepiphyseal dysplasia congenita (known simply as SEDc, or SED) — often have to undergo numerous orthopedic surgeries from infancy on. Some can only walk short distances, using crutches, scooters, and wheelchairs to get around.

So, yes, dwarfism, even achondroplastic dwarfism, is a disability, and not just a socially constructed one. But it's a difference, too, and many within the community take great pride in that difference. Ruth Ricker, an achondroplastic dwarf and a past president of Little People of America, goes so far as to say that though she would like to see medical advances eliminate the complications of dwarfism, she would object to the elimination of the short stature that is its most obvious characteristic. "To change the dwarfism itself, as in the height — I think it would be hard for many of us, psychologically, to say we'd do that, because it's so intertwined with what makes us *us*," she once told me. "It would deny an integral part of myself that I have some pride in. It could be the end of achondroplasia."

Thus the answer to the "defect or difference?" conundrum is: both. Each of us has something like thirty thousand genes, and random mutations are not uncommon. It's just that the effects of the mutation that causes dwarfism are so obvious. As with the genetic difference that causes one person's eyes to be brown and another's blue, the mutation that causes dwarfism says nothing important about the individual who has it. But as with the genetic difference that causes Down syndrome, or Lou Gehrig's disease, it is indeed, a mistake, an error, a cosmic typo imprinted on each of the many billions of cells that the average human body contains.

Once, someone posted a message to the Dwarfism List saying

something to the effect of *I am not a mistake* — a variation of "God doesn't make mistakes." Someone else posted a response that I think got perfectly at the difference/defect divide. I'm paraphrasing, but it went pretty much like this: *Of course you're not a mistake. People aren't mistakes. On the other hand, genomes can contain mistakes, and dwarfism is clearly a mistake. But we are all more than the sum of our genomes.*

Becky recovered quickly from the meconium and hypoglycemia and came home within a few days of delivery. We received final word on her condition shortly thereafter. Barbara and I were summoned to our pediatrician's office, where we were given a brief overview of achondroplasia and a pamphlet assuring us that Becky would likely enjoy a reasonably normal life. I mainly just looked at the photos in the pamphlet of dwarf kids and adults and tried to imagine how Becky would fit into those pictures. We were also offered psychological counseling, which we turned down, and an appointment with the geneticist, which we accepted.

Some people report having a hard time adjusting to their child's dwarfism. I certainly can understand that. But for Barbara and me, the fall of 1992 wasn't a time of terrible angst, anxiety, or recriminations. We talked about this strange new reality that had been introduced into our lives, but we had no idea of what to expect. And in our ignorance, we chose to believe that Becky would be fine — just really, really short.

In part, I attribute this to the positive picture that had been painted for us by Becky's doctors, a picture very different from what would have been offered us a generation earlier, when parents were often informed that their dwarf children might be mentally retarded and would likely not live long. Soon after Becky had been diagnosed, I looked up achondroplasia in the *Encyclopedia Britannica* at our town library — and was shocked to read that many children die during their first year. But the encyclopedia was ancient; in any case, it was so out of sync with what we had been told, and with what I wanted to believe, that I just put it out of my mind. In part, too, I attribute my outlook to the depression I had recently recovered from. Feeling like I'd only just made it to the other side, I was determined not to slide back. Barbara, focused on the task at hand, was concerned about Becky's future, but was far more wrapped up in taking care of her baby's needs. Becky appeared to be fine, Timmy was doing great, so why worry?

I've read and heard stories about parents who actually go through a phenomenon that Joan Ablon and others refer to as *mourning the loss of the perfect child.* But that really doesn't get at what we were going through that fall. It just wasn't that dramatic. If Becky's physical differences were more obvious, if her disabilities were more serious, if her ability to think and to love were at issue, things might have been different. Barbara says she mourned, but for Becky rather than for herself — for the discrimination she knew she'd encounter one day, for the stares and giggles and teasing that were sure to come. One of Barbara's high-school classmates was a dwarf, and they'd worked together on a studentrun television newscast. So Barbara had more-concrete knowledge than I of the difficulties that dwarfs must face.

But as I would soon learn, my *idea* of dwarfism did not match the *reality* of dwarfism. I wasn't ready yet, but I was about to begin my real education in what it means to be a dwarf. It's an education that will never be finished, and that will always be hindered by the fact that, as an average-size father, I'm on the outside looking in. But at least I began to realize what I didn't know — and that what I didn't know could kill my little girl.

For Barbara and me, naming our daughter Rebecca Elizabeth was an act of affirmation. We had decided on that name sometime earlier for our baby if it turned out to be a girl. There was no special significance to "Rebecca;" we just liked it. "Elizabeth" is the middle name of Barbara's sister, Mary. When Becky was born, we went ahead and named her Rebecca Elizabeth without so much as a discussion. We were not going to save it for a future daughter with less-uncertain prospects. We were sending a signal — to ourselves as much as anyone — that this *was* the daughter we'd always wanted.

But the daughter we'd always wanted was beginning to have problems, big problems — far bigger than we realized until it was almost too late. Becky was a content and happy infant, smiley and engaged, easier than Tim had been at that age, but also more fragile. The outsize dimensions of her head, her weak neck, and her poor muscle tone gave her a floppy quality, and she had to be held *just so* lest she be hurt. And that was the least of it. She had a perpetual cold, and, since she couldn't breathe through her nose very well, she couldn't breast-feed with much success. Barbara had to give up when Becky was around four months old. At night, in her crib, the top of her head would break into a cold sweat. She'd arch her neck way, way back, as though she were trying to find a position where she could get enough air in her lungs — which, we later found out, was exactly what she was doing. Her pediatrician, Dr. Robert Krachman, tried several antibiotics, none of which seemed to do any good. He x-rayed her lungs and found that they were clear — something he couldn't explain, given that she sounded like she was congested. Finally, and to his everlasting credit, he threw up his hands and suggested that Becky see a specialist.

Once a month, Dr. Daniel Shannon, a pediatric pulmonary specialist at Boston's Massachusetts General Hospital and a leading authority in his field, would travel fifteen miles north to Beverly Hospital, where he would see patients in a clinical setting. Barbara took Becky to see Dr. Shannon in January. As Barbara described it, he took one look at Becky, one look at the results of a blood test she'd had done prior to the clinic, and said she almost certainly need a tracheostomy. Her respiratory system, he explained, was so tiny that she was unable to expel carbon dioxide as efficiently as she should. As a result, the CO2 was rising to dangerous levels in her blood. Her heart, brain, and lungs could be damaged; she could even die if she caught a cold. Becky's problems were not so acute that she needed to be hospitalized immediately, but he recommended a follow-up within the next several weeks.

That follow-up never took place. On a bitterly cold Saturday night in February, we took the kids to the mall just to get out of the house and hang out for a while. Timmy enjoyed running around a toy store. Becky alternated between the carriage and Barbara's arms. We ran into a friend and talked, getting home later than we had wanted. Becky had yet another cold and was exhausted. So were we all. The next morning Becky seemed to be filling up again, so Barbara took her to the "urgent care" department of the clinic that our HMO ran. They gave her a quick exam and told Barbara to get her to Mass General as soon as possible. She drove to Boston and took Becky to the emergency room; from there, Becky was admitted to the pediatric intensive-care unit (PICU). The diagnosis: respiratory syncytial virus, or RSV.

Now, in most kids, RSV causes nothing more than an unusually bad cold. It's potentially serious; according to the Centers for Disease Control and Prevention, it causes infections of both the upper and lower respiratory tracts, and can lead to pneumonia. But nearly all children get RSV at some point, and nearly all of them come out of it fine. In Becky's case, though, the copious amounts of mucus that RSV produces clogged airways that, because of her dwarfism, were already so tiny that she couldn't breathe as efficiently as her body required. Now her blood was both starved for oxygen and loaded with carbon dioxide. Her life was in danger.

RSV is perilous to any child who's younger than six months. Another baby in the PICU, a girl, had to be put into a chemically induced coma so that doctors could force a respirator down her throat. Becky was sick, very sick; but she proved to be a tough little kid, and she began to rally before Dr. Shannon had to do anything quite so drastic. Barbara was at Becky's side almost constantly. I had driven Tim to Albany to stay with Barbara's sister, Mary Zysinski, so that I could spend most of my non-working hours in the PICU, too. We were in a weird state of limbo, a bubble almost. The PICU is an alternate universe; at any time of the day or night it is as bright as noon, with nurses and doctors rushing about. All around us, kids were desperately ill. One little boy died after his liver transplant failed. Others hovered somewhere between life and death. To a certain extent we were removed from that. Becky, though a long way from well, was in no immediate danger; she mainly needed to be monitored closely while we figured out the next step. Whenever I visited, I experienced a combination of anxiety over Becky's condition and guilt over how much worse the other parents had it. I felt like an interloper. Yet there was no question that Becky was where she needed to be.

During the next few weeks Becky kept improving. But the level of oxygen in her blood remained too low, and the CO2 remained too high, even though she was getting extra oxygen through a tube under her nose. It wasn't just that her airways were too small; it's that, when she slept, her trachea would nearly close, creating an obstruction, which, in turn, caused sleep apnea. Other characteristics of achondroplasia combined to worsen her breathing difficulties. Her ribcage was small, which meant that her lungs couldn't inflate fully. Her face was (and is) unusually flat, giving her tiny sinuses that easily become congested. An MRI was taken to make sure that Becky's foramen magnum — that is, the top of the spinal column, where it meets the skull — was not pinching and squeezing her brain stem, a rare but by no means unheard-of problem for kids with achondroplasia. Such a complication can also cause apnea, thus mimicking some of Becky's symptoms. It was a tight fit, as it is with all achon kids, but it wasn't *too* tight. She wouldn't need spinal surgery. Still, a tracheostomy loomed as increasingly likely.

I didn't doubt that Dr. Shannon knew what he was doing, and it was of no small significance that he'd told us he had some experience in treating dwarfs. But Becky's life and future were at stake, and I wanted to know more before agreeing to a trach. I dug out the material on Little People of America that the geneticist had given us. The phone numbers and contact information were out of date, but one call led to another until, finally, I was put in touch with Ruth Ricker, at that time LPA's senior vice president, who, I learned, lived in Boston, barely a block from the *Phoenix*'s offices. She agreed to pay us a visit. On a Saturday morning, a few hours before our daily trek back to the hospital, she pulled into our driveway and jumped out — down would be more accurate — carrying a bag of muffins and waddling toward our back door. Ruth stands a shade under four feet, at least a half-foot shorter than what I'd expected.

The experience was disconcerting, but it gave us reason to hope, too. We learned that Ruth, like Barbara and me, had gone to Northeastern; that she held an important job in the civil-rights division of the U.S. Department of Education; and that, like us, she followed the Red Sox and politics. From all appearances, Ruth had the kind of life we wanted for Becky. Here was proof that it was possible. If only we could get her well.

Ruth also brought something of more immediate importance: a recommendation that we contact Dr. Cheryl Reid, a pulmonary specialist from New Jersey who was a member of LPA's medical-advisory board, a group of physicians who specialize in treating the complications of dwarfism. Dr. Shannon was agitating for us to make a decision on the tracheostomy; Barbara was ready, I wasn't. I contacted Dr. Reid, and sent all of Becky's records to her after she agreed to review them. Several days later, she gave me the second-best news I could have heard: that Dr. Shannon knew exactly what he was doing, and that we should proceed with the trach. (The best news, of course, would have been that Becky didn't need a trach, and that we should get her away from that nut Shannon ASAP.)

The surgery was scheduled, then postponed when Becky caught a bug unrelated to the RSV. Finally, on the afternoon of Friday, February 26, 1993, Becky was wheeled into the operating room. The operation was performed by Dr. Michael Cunningham, an ear-nose-and-throat specialist at the Massachusetts Eye and Ear Infirmary, which is affiliated with Mass General. I was scared, anxious to the point of lightheadedness; Barbara was outwardly calm, inwardly in agony. And our feelings were only amplified by what was going on around us. Terrorists had attacked the World Trade Center for the first time that afternoon, and we watched CNN in the waiting room as the injured were led to safety. Closer at hand, immediately after Becky's surgery we and other anxious parents were shooed out of the recovery room to make way for a young gunshot victim; he later died, as I recall.

Amid this chaos, Becky's surgery went well. But seeing her afterward was a shock. A tube was emanating from a freshly cut hole in her throat, which was in turn connected to a hose that led to a CPAP machine ("CPAP" stands for "continuous positive airway pressure"), a loud, monstrous-looking device that made it easier for her to breathe while she was adjusting to the drastic change in her respiratory system. The sight of our beautiful baby in such a state was emotionally overwhelming. I was numb; I looked, but I'm not sure I saw, or believed.

Meanwhile, we worried about the effect this was all having on Tim. When I'd brought him to Albany, I was sure he'd be there only a week. He was two years old, just learning to talk, and absolutely thrived on attention from his parents. At the end of that first week, when we realized we weren't ready for him to come home yet, I drove to Albany to spend the day with him. He was overwrought and threw an eleven-on-a-scale-of-ten tantrum at McDonald's, behavior that was very unlike him. That night, driving back on the Massachusetts Turnpike, it began to snow, hard, and my car, a seven-year-old Corolla, sputtered out. I pulled over into the breakdown lane in some nether region between Springfield and Worcester, cursing, thankful only that Tim wasn't with me. This was the pre-cellphone era, and not a state-police cruiser was to be seen. To my grateful astonishment, I was able to restart the car after about a half-hour, and from there eased it to Mass General for a late-night visit with Becky and Barbara. After another week, it was clear that Becky's hospital stay was going to be a long one and, since Tim couldn't stay in Albany forever, I brought him home. Mainly, he stayed with friends and neighbors, but at least he got to spend some time with us.

Becky was in the PICU a total of five weeks — three before her surgery, two after — followed by three weeks on a regular pediatric floor. She was gradually weaned off the CPAP machine, though she continued to need oxygen. Eventually, her personality began to reemerge, but there were aspects of the new Becky that were unnerving — none more so than her inability to make herself heard. With the trach, air was circumventing Becky's vocal cords, so even if she tried to make a sound, all that came out was a hiss. She laughed silently. She cried silently.

So did we.

During this time, the hospital staff began preparing us for the responsibility of caring for a baby with a tracheostomy, which, we were about to learn, was fairly daunting. We didn't know how long Becky would even have the trach — two years was the best guess, though Dr. Reid had warned me that it could go on much longer than that. But we did know that Becky's care was going to be phenomenally expensive, and that our HMO wouldn't pay the full freight. It's ironic. Not that many years earlier, we were told, babies with trachs were automatically sent to chronic-care hospitals, running up catastrophic bills that were routinely paid for by insurance companies. At some point someone wised up and said, *Wait a minute. These kids can be cared for more cheaply, and will do much better, if they're sent home. All they need is some nursing care and some equipment.* But home nurses are not routinely covered by private medical insurance. So I was dispatched to our local welfare office for the sole purpose of submitting a Medicaid application that was certain to be rejected because of our middle-class income. After that, we could apply for a special state program that covered home health care. Our insurance company would foot the bills until then.

There was more, much more. Barbara and I met with a nurse at Mass General who showed us how to change Becky's trach tube, how to suction it if it became clogged with mucus, and how to yank it out if there were an emergency. I was there, but I wasn't; I kind of zoned out, watching and listening, but telling myself I would never be able to do that. And I was right, sort of. Other than learning how to use the suction machine to remove phlegm from her trach tube — an absolute necessity if I were to be with Becky for more than fifteen minutes — I kept myself at a safe remove from trach care, never changing or cleaning her tube or changing or even tying the shoelace-like straps that held it in place. Oh, I would help occasionally, but I was more than happy to let Barbara take the lead and pass it off to whichever home nurse was on duty if Barbara wasn't around. For some reason I never felt competent enough to take charge, and was always afraid I would do something wrong, something to impede Becky's breathing, something that would hurt her. It wasn't rational or even particularly responsible. But I convinced myself that it was the best I could manage.

In early April, eight weeks after she'd checked in to the Mass General emergency room, Becky was ready to come home. We have a photo of her in her hospital room that day, strapped into one of those infant car seats that can be carried by a handle (not good for dwarfs because it scrunches their backs, but we didn't know), a big smile on her face, a bluish plastic hose running from her trach to a portable oxygen tank. And we headed home, uncertain of the future, and of our ability to handle whatever that future was going to bring.

Chapter Three

Just Like Tom Thumb's Blues

On an unseasonably cold March morning, many years after Becky's precarious start had given way to a blissfully uneventful childhood, I drove to the Middleborough Historical Museum, which consists of two small red houses just outside the downtown of the small town in southeastern Massachusetts from which it takes its name. I'd grown up in Middleborough and had visited the museum any number of times during my childhood. As kids, we had called it the Tom Thumb Museum because of its display of memorabilia on the lives of Charles Stratton — a.k.a. Tom Thumb — and his wife, Lavinia Warren, who is Middleborough's best-known native daughter. I had come to see it again, for the first time in probably thirty-five years, not as a child marveling over the two tiny folk, but as the father of a dwarf, both curious about and repelled by the notion of little people being put on public display.

Gladys Beals, a thin, gray-haired elderly woman with a friendly and welcoming manner, was waiting for me. The museum operates on such a shoestring that it is open only from July through October. During the other eight months you have to make an appointment. The building was unheated and cold enough that we could see our breath. Mrs. Beals led me through three rooms devoted to General and Mrs. Tom Thumb. She pointed out such artifacts as a photograph of the mansion that the Strattons had built in Middleborough (still lived in, though long since retrofitted for average-size occupants), a black gown that Lavinia wore to an audience with Queen Victoria, books, gloves, shoes, roller skates, and a stereoscope with a three-dimensional photo of their wedding in New York City, one of the premier social events of the 1860s.

Mrs. Beals explained that she had become interested in Charles and Lavinia during the thirteen years that her late husband, Robert, had been head of the historical society. "We became so enamored of the little people," she said. "When we came in, we said, 'Hi, kids,' and when we left, we'd say, 'Bye, kids.'" She made it clear that she admired the Strattons, and she emphatically defended P. T. Barnum, the legendary nineteenth-century showman, against charges that he exploited his two most popular attractions. "He did it in a very, very fair manner," she said. (That does, in fact, appear to be the case. By all accounts, the Strattons shrewdly exploited themselves, and Barnum gave them the means by which to do it.) Mrs. Beals saw nothing wrong with the Strattons' making a public spectacle of their physical difference in order to earn a living. During my own childhood visits to the museum, it had never occurred to me that there might be something wrong with it either. Of course, that was a good twenty-five years before Becky's birth raised philosophical issues for me that most people never have a reason to think about.

The Strattons represented the pinnacle of a time when dwarfs were treated as public curiosities, as wonders of nature. And though this phenomenon has not disappeared entirely, today we have a very different attitude toward dwarfism. We recognize it as a medical condition and consider it to be either a genetic flaw or a difference worthy of recognition and protection, like race or sexual orientation. People still stare, of course, as they stared at Becky during our Labor Day trip to Story Land. The difference is that today the stare is directed not at a person on display, but rather — or so I hope — at someone trying to go about her business just like anyone else.

Among the first recorded examples of a dwarf being put on display for the amusement of the paying public was that of an anonymous Dutchman, who was observed in 1581 by the English tailor and antiquarian John Stow and described in his *Chronicles of England.* As recounted by Hy Roth and Robert Cromie in their 1980 book, *The Little People,* the dwarf, who was three feet tall, was displayed in London alongside a seven-foot-seven giant. The larger man was hobbled by a stunt gone bad, having broken both legs in the course of lifting a full beer barrel. The dwarf, who was also lame, performed such tricks as dancing and walking upright between the giant's legs, feathered hat and all.

It was within this dubious tradition that Charles Sherwood Stratton and Mercy Lavinia Warren Bump Stratton Magri launched their oddly spectacular careers.

Charles Stratton was born on January 4, 1838, in Bridgeport, Connecticut, to parents of average height — or, as an 1863 pamphlet on the Strattons' marriage put it, "His parents were persons about whom there existed no peculiarity, either in mental or physical organization." His mother attributed her son's dwarfism to the grief she had experienced when the family dog died during her pregnancy.

Charles never had a say over the direction his life would take. When he was just five years old, his parents allowed another son of Bridgeport, P. T. Barnum, to take him to New York City and put him on display at his American Museum. The museum showed everything from middlebrow plays for family audiences — Barnum went so far as to edit the sex out of Shakespeare — to such oddities as a "mermaid" consisting of a monkey's head sewn onto a fish's body. Barnum changed Charles's age from five to eleven in order to exaggerate his short stature, gave him the name Tom Thumb after a legendary member of King Arthur's roundtable, and trained him to do such tricks as imitating Napoleon and engaging in mock battle, with Barnum as Goliath and Stratton as David.

Stratton was two-foot-eleven at the age of twenty-five, but grew slightly more as he got older. His dwarfism was most likely caused by growth-hormone deficiency — that is, his body did not produce enough natural growth hormone for him to reach his full height. Such dwarfs, whose limbs are in the same proportion to the rest of their bodies as those of an average-size person's, were prized in the entertainment business, since their appearance was thought to be more pleasing than that of, say, an achondroplastic dwarf. "As symmetrical as an Apollo," Barnum once said admiringly of his prodigy.

Stratton was an enormous hit with the public, so much so that he secured Barnum's reputation and fortune. In 1844 Stratton and his mentor traveled to London, where he was presented to Queen Victoria ("How d'ye do," he said to her) and amused the court by becoming involved in an altercation with one of the royal poodles, memorably depicted in a drawing done at the time. From there he traveled throughout Europe, occasionally making use of an ornate miniature carriage pulled by ponies. When he returned to New York, in 1847, his appearances at the American Museum broke attendance records.

If Stratton's parents set their son's destiny before he was old enough to have a say in the matter, the opposite was true of his future wife. She was born on October 31, 1842, in Middleborough, to the long-established and prosperous Bumps, a family that traces its roots to the *Mayflower* and is well known in the town to this day. Her full name was Mercy Lavinia Warren Bump. Like Charles, Lavinia was apparently growthhormone deficient. She stopped growing at the age of ten, when she was two-foot-ten. In an unusually progressive move for its day, the town's school committee hired her to teach elementary school when she turned sixteen. In a series of autobiographical essays that she wrote for the *New York Tribune Sunday Magazine* in 1906, she recalled the joy and dedication she brought to that task:

> I was very zealous in my duty, and at the end of the term received the commendation and thanks of the committee for the excellent discipline I maintained, as well as the progress made by the pupils under my tuition. The youngest even was far above me in stature, yet all seemed anxious to be obedient and to please me.

Yet when a cousin suggested that she join his "floating palace of curiosities" on the Ohio and Mississippi Rivers, she agreed, apparently without hesitation. As she writes of her erstwhile teaching career, "I thought I had now found a proper and genial vocation, but during the subsequent vacation an event occurred which entirely changed the tenor of my life." From there, it was a very short leap to P. T. Barnum's revue.

Lavinia's career choice shows why it's intellectually hazardous to judge Barnum and his ilk by the standards of our time. As Gladys Beals insisted, quite rightly, Barnum didn't exploit the Strattons, because they did exactly what they wanted to do — particularly Lavinia, who, unlike Charles, joined Barnum's troupe as an adult. Lavinia gave up a promising career as a teacher, in a community where she and her family were respected, in order to join a freak show. The Strattons made a lot of money and lived well, denying themselves nothing. It wasn't Barnum's fault that they ended up blowing most of their fortune — after all, he was pretty good at blowing fortunes in his own right. Indeed, at one point, after a fire had consumed the American Museum, Charles Stratton came out of semiretirement to go on tour with Barnum, helping his old boss raise money for no reasons other than loyalty and affection. Criticizing Barnum for displaying dwarfs, along with "armless wonders," microcephalics (dubbed "Aztecs" for some reason), Siamese twins, and other human curiosities, is like criticizing George Washington and Thomas Jefferson for keeping slaves. Such criticism is not so much valid or invalid as it is ahistorical.

Barnum dropped the harsh-sounding "Bump" from his new star's name, and she was known as Lavinia Warren from that point on. Her 1863 marriage to Charles Stratton at Grace Church in New York was one of the great media spectacles of the era, with two thousand people attending and gifts coming in from the likes of the Astors, the Vanderbilts, and President and Mrs. Lincoln, who received the couple at the White House during their honeymoon tour. The attendants were two other Barnum dwarfs: "Commodore" George Washington Morrison Nutt, an earlier suitor of Lavinia's, and her sister Huldah Pierce Bump, known as Minnie Warren. Months later, the proud husband and wife were photographed posing with a baby — a hoax aimed at keeping interest alive in the Strattons, as well as feeding curiosity about their sex lives. It was a hoax they could not sustain, and, after a discreet interval, it was announced that the baby had died of a brain inflammation.

Hard times lay ahead. Charles, who enjoyed cigars and rich food, died of a stroke in 1883. Lavinia, strapped for cash, married another dwarf, "Count" Primo Magri; along with his brother, "Baron" Ernesto Magri, they formed the Lilliputian Opera Company, hit the road, and enjoyed some success. But Lavinia could never reconcile her spending with her income, and there was far less public interest in her as a plump, elderly dwarf than there had been when she was young and attractive. She and Primo opened a general store in Middleborough; they also for a time became the best-known residents of something called "Midget City," at Coney Island, one of a number of such theme parks to spring up around the country. Lavinia died in 1919, and was buried in Bridgeport alongside Charles.

Don't shed any tears for the Strattons. They lived the life they chose, and by all appearances they lived it well. But as the historian

Robert Bogdan points out, the tragedy of Charles and Lavinia Stratton was that they lived a lie and convinced themselves that it was the truth. The Strattons were intelligent, normal, average people in every way except for their short stature. Yet they believed what they were constantly told: that they were exceptional performers, artists, entitled to the accolades and gifts that came their way, even though they were, in reality, mediocre talents whose only real attraction was their unusual appearance. They were exhibited in what Bogdan calls the "high aggrandized mode," depicted as people of refinement and gentility. It was mostly farce, but as they got older, they ceased to see the farce.

"Tom Thumb became a serious Charles Stratton, a person who wanted others to respect him because of what he had achieved and to ignore how he might have achieved it, the basis of his fame," Bogdan writes. In fact, the lives that they enjoyed were not just dependent on the mere fact that they were dwarfs, but that they were a *certain type* of dwarf, "perfect humans in miniature," to use another of Barnum's phrases. Had they been disproportionate, they never would have been dressed up in tuxedos and flowing gowns. More likely they would have been cast as clowns or freaks, or as "Esquimaux" (Eskimos), dressed in furs against a backdrop of fake icebergs, like an achondroplastic dwarf known as Miss Olaf Krarer. That the Strattons' particular accident of birth turned out in their favor made it no less accidental.

In walking through the Middleborough museum, I found it difficult to reconcile nineteenth-century attitudes with twenty-first-century sensibilities — especially since the attitudes that were reflected in those displays were so at odds with what I want, and expect, for Becky.

So my favorite exhibit turned out to be something that spoke not of its time, but of any time. It was a photograph of Lavinia, Primo, and Ernesto, somewhat advanced in years, sitting around a dining-room table with three average-size adults — Lavinia's brothers, perhaps — in the dark, Victorianstyle Bump family home. There was a certain quality to the photo that at first I couldn't put my finger on. Later I realized that it was its simple portrayal of normal family life, away from the spotlight, unself-conscious, the three dwarfs composing themselves to be photographed not as curiosities but for the same reason that any of us pose for a camera-wielding brother or aunt.

In that photograph, I could see Lavinia Warren not as a world-famous oddity, but rather as the proper Middleborough schoolteacher that she was and might have continued to be.

The first dwarf whom researchers know anything about was a young man who died more than eleven thousand years ago in southern Italy. His grave was unearthed in 1963, but it wasn't until 1987 that a group of anthropologists, led by David Frayer of the University of Kansas, studied his skeleton and reported on its significance in the journal *Nature*. According to Frayer, the young man appeared to be about seventeen years old and less than four feet tall. Although humans at that time had to contend with the severe, subsistence-level existence of the Ice Age, foraging for food and living in caves, the young man appeared to have been well cared for, and to have been treated as a valued member of his clan. At burial he was wrapped in the arms of a thirty-five-year-old average-size woman whom the investigators guessed may have been his mother.

The man's dwarfism type was identified as acromesomelic dysplasia, a rare disorder that is similar in appearance to achondroplasia except those who have it tend to be a few inches shorter. Anthropologists disagree as to whether the clan's acceptance of a dwarf was evidence of empathy or of his ability to adapt and contribute despite his disability. My betting is on the latter. Though he was probably exempted from having to spear woolly mammoths, he could have held his own at other tasks because acromesomelic dysplasia usually carries with it few health complications, fewer even than achondroplasia. As the Smithsonian Institution's Donald Ortner told *Scientific American*, "Certainly some support mechanism had to be there. But it's quite remarkable how capable people are at adapting to physical disabilities of one sort or another."

Dwarfs played a special role in the court and religious life of ancient Egypt, some four thousand to five thousand years ago. The scholar Bonnie Sampsell writes that dwarfs served the pharoah in such positions as "personal attendant in elite households, supervisor of clothing and linen, pet handler, jewelry maker and entertainer or dancer." Achondroplastic dwarfs were often the subjects of statues and carvings, sometimes with the facial and limb characteristics of achondroplasia toned down and stylized, sometimes portrayed with perfect realism.

The most fascinating of these Egyptian dwarfs was Seneb, whose *mastaba*, or tomb, was excavated in 1927. Sampsell writes that inscriptions on the tomb show Seneb held such positions as "Director of Dwarfs in Charge of Dressing," "Director of Weaving in the Palace," and "Great One of the Sedan Chair" — possibly a reference to the chair of the pharoah himself. Seneb, who lived in approximately 2300 B.C., was also a priest. Seneb's most striking legacy is a beautifully painted statue of him, his wife, Senetites, and their son and daughter. Seneb and Senetites are sitting on a slab; Senetites is average-size, and her legs dangle over, her feet resting on the floor below and her hand affectionately touching her husband's arm. Seneb sits cross-legged on top of the slab, his short arms folded in front of him, his head slightly larger than his wife's. To fill in the space next to Senetites's legs, the sculptor added carvings of their son and daughter. It is a remarkable piece of art, not just for its stunning execution, but for the sense of easy normality it imparts to a dwarf husband and his average-size wife, a relationship that would draw stares today, let alone more than four thousand years ago.

Some Egyptian gods also seem to have been portrayed as dwarfs, such as Ptah-Pataikos and Bes — the latter of whom, Sampsell writes, was thought to protect the bodies of the dead and to keep diseases, dangerous animals, and evil spirits away from the living. (I say "seem" because Sampsell notes that Bes was also part animal, which calls into question whether his dwarf-like features were actually intended as such.) "In probably no other culture," Sampsell says, "have dwarfs been given a more visible role and apparently a chance to enjoy a normal life than in the Old Kingdom of ancient Egypt." That's a bold assertion on the basis of scant archeological evidence, but the benign countenances of Seneb and Senetites suggest that the ancient Egyptians could teach us a few things about accepting — and even celebrating — diversity. Certainly the same could not be said of all ancient peoples. Consider the Book of Leviticus, in which God himself forbade dwarfs — not to mention anyone who was blind, lame, deformed, had scabs, or had even suffered a ruptured testicle — from serving at his altar, lest they "profane . . . my sanctuaries."

Throughout history, dwarfs have played roles separate and apart, both high and low, from valued advisers to pets or jesters. According to the anthropologist Francis Johnston, dwarfs were kept by the Roman emperors Tiberius, Alexander Severus, and Mark Antony, sometimes as counselors, sometimes as mere decoration. Dwarfs were also forced to fight as gladiators in the Colosseum.

An unusually detailed history of dwarfs is offered by Hy Roth and Robert Cromie in *The Little People.* Their presentation raises questions — the book is filled with photographs of dwarfs in offbeat and often-demeaning entertainment roles, and the foreword, by Irving Wallace, begins unpromisingly, "This is a wonderful big book about a mad assortment of little people." Still, Roth and Cromie appear to have done their homework. They are particularly good on the role of dwarfs in Western mythology: the mine dwarfs of England, who could kill miners by causing the roof to collapse, the shaft to explode, or water to rush in unless they were bribed with food and other gifts; the "Black Dwarf," a curmudgeonly hermit who inspired Sir Walter Scott; the Teutonic dwarfs, skilled swordmakers who, when angered, stole crops and children, and who were created from grubs found in the decaying body of a giant; trolls, who hated noise; elves, who danced in the moonlight; and on and on it goes.

As for actual historical figures, Attila the Hun is sometimes described as having been a dwarf, although Roth and Cromie caution that little is known about him. Most likely references to Attila's possible dwarfism survive because it's included in Gibbon's *The History of the Decline and Fall of the Roman Empire*, which in turn relied on ancient works of dubious accuracy. The *Lancet* published an article in 1991 suggesting that Richard III was a dwarf. St. Gregory of Tours is sometimes described as having been a dwarf, though that claim, like the one regarding Attila, is considered unlikely by experts today.

Among the most famous dwarfs was the Englishman Jeffrey Hudson (1619-1682), who was introduced to Queen Henrietta Maria when he popped out of a cold pie that had been brought to her. Hudson's biographer Nick Page describes the mindset of the seventeenth-century court of Charles I this way: "A dwarf, a tiny boy only eighteen inches high. What better present for the Queen with her monkeys and dogs than a little human, all of her own?" (The extent of Hudson's short stature was almost certainly exaggerated.) Hudson did enough living for several lives. He was named a captain for the royalist side in the English Civil War; he shot and killed a man in a duel; and he was captured by the Barbary pirates twice — the second occasion resulting in more than two decades in slavery in North Africa, during which time he allegedly added nearly two feet to his foot-and-a-half-high stature, apparently the result of his pituitary system's belatedly kicking in.

A French dwarf by the name of Richebourg, said to be somewhere between twenty-three-and-a-half and thirty-three-and-a-half inches tall, was an aide to the Duchesse d'Orléans, mother of Louis Philippe, the future King of the French. Richebourg's claim to fame was his role as a surreptitious courier during the French Revolution. "The device," Roth and Cromie write, "was simple: Richebourg, dressed in a baby's outfit, was carried by a nursemaid with the papers concealed in his clothing."

Until the modern era, no one did more to imbue dwarfs with a sense of dignity and humanity than the seventeenthcentury Spanish-court artist Diego Velázquez. To do so, Velázquez had both to adopt and rise above the standards of his day. As the art critic Norbert Wolf writes,

> In Spain (and other countries, too), there was a long tradition of including dwarfs in royal portraits as subordinate figures. Basically, these deformed little creatures were merely attributes of royal dignity, part of the furnishings of the court and regarded as neuter beings rather than fully human. Velázquez accepts this distinction, yet ultimately he cancels it out.

As an example of this duality, Wolf offers *Prince Baltasar Carlos with a Dwarf* (1631), in which the sixteen-month-old prince is shown with a young female dwarf in a dark green dress. She is clearly subordinate, and Velázquez paints her in darker, broader brushstrokes than he does his royal subject. Yet, somehow, he manages to depict the girl with more realism and humanity than her playmate. As Wolf writes, "the melancholy inherent in the picturesque shadows says more about the dwarf girl's destiny than the bright flesh tints of Baltasar Carlos's face can tell us about his radiant, princely figure."

Dwarfs were also depicted in Velázquez's masterpiece, *Las Meninas* (1656-57), a surrealistic treatment of the Infanta Margarita and the rest of the royal family that anticipated Salvador Dal' by three centuries. A central figure in *Las Meninas* is Velázquez himself, caught in the act of painting. In the foreground, on the right-hand side of the canvas, are a female dwarf, Mari-Bárbola, and a male dwarf, Nicolasico Pertusato, who rests his foot on an enormous dog.

Among the more notable aspects of the painting is Velázquez's sympathetic portrayal of Mari-Bárbola, whose gaze evenly meets that of the viewer, straightforward and unashamed. So I was stunned by Wolf's description of her as "grotesquely misshapen." To me, her looks are pretty much standard achon; her facial figures appear to be more affected by achondroplasia than is typical, but she is hardly grotesque, or even particularly unattractive. And unlike Wolf's earlier description of dwarfs as "deformed little creatures," when he was writing about seventeenth-century attitudes, this time he is speaking for himself.

Is this how the world sees Rebecca Elizabeth Kennedy? As "grotesquely misshapen"? Is that why strangers stare and point and whisper? Just as I can't imagine why Norbert Wolf finds Mari-Bárbola's face so repulsive, I can't imagine what people are thinking when they stare at my daughter. Or why anyone would pay money to stare at another human being. But it happened. It happens still, under the guise of "dwarf tossing" or "midget wrestling." The roots of such spectacles are deep and apparently not easily eradicated. They say much about cultural attitudes toward difference. Rather than seeing dwarfism as one of many attributes of a person, dwarfism is seen *as* the person: he is a dwarf, not a person. That's why some people within the dwarf community would rather talk about *persons with dwarfism* rather than *dwarfs*. To substitute the difference for the person is to deny his humanity. It's an old story, and a current one, too.

Barbara and I think Becky is beautiful. To those who don't know her, though, her size and disproportionate appearance are the first things they notice. Achondroplasia? What's that? For many people, she's the first dwarf they've ever seen — maybe the only one they'll *ever* see outside of a media context. Most people never have the opportunity to assimilate dwarfs into their consciousness the way they have assimilated, say, people of different racial backgrounds. To them, dwarfs will always look funny, or wrong, because they're never going to see enough dwarfs to register them as just another type of normal. Three days at a Little People of America conference and they'd get over it. But unless they have a family member who's a dwarf, that's probably not going to happen.

Documentaries on dwarfs appear regularly on the Discovery Channel, HBO, even MTV. Sally Jessy Raphael, Maury Povich, Montel Williams, and other TV talk-show hosts frequently have dwarfs on as guests. Howard Stern puts on the air such sorry cases as "Hank the Angry, Drunken Dwarf," who died in 2001 from complications related to alcohol abuse, and "Beetlejuice," an African-American dwarf who makes a fool of himself by pretending (or maybe not) to be mentally disabled. Somewhere in the deep recesses of our collective psyche, we haven't evolved much past the delight that Henrietta Maria felt when young Jeffrey Hudson popped out of her pie.

Recently, the public has been captivated by a commercial for

Apple Computer starring "Mini-Me," Verne Troyer, the two-foot-eight actor from the *Austin Powers* movies, and Yao Ming, the seven-foot-five center for the Houston Rockets. Yao's role is to make you gasp; Troyer's, to make you laugh — as, in fact, Yao does when Troyer pulls out a big-as-he-is Macintosh PowerBook. It's an entertaining ad, and Troyer's non-stereotypical role as an airline passenger, perhaps a businessman, is something of a step forward. But the humor depends on our having internalized a stereotype about who is automatically entitled to respect and who must earn it — in this case, by whipping out the biggest, uh, laptop on the planet.

"We seem to be a fad," says Hillary Melechen, a woman with achondroplasia from St. Louis, Missouri. I'd met Melechen at a screening of *Liebe Perla*, a documentary about a family of Hungarian-Jewish dwarfs who survived Auschwitz only because the infamous Josef Mengele had saved them for his experiments. Melechen had said some interesting things about being both a dwarf and a Jew, and so I sought her out later to ask her about our cultural fascination with dwarfs.

"I don't know," she told me, but she quickly warmed to the subject. "I think it's — I wonder if it's partly because difference is so uncomfortable in this culture. And we're an easy target. We're so few. It's a difference that's so looks-based, and we do so much in this culture based on looks." She added: "We are disturbing to people to look at. When I was a kid, there were people who saw me and they'd scream."

They'd scream? Sitting before me was an attractive, thoughtful forty-three-year-old woman with blond frizzy hair and wire-rimmed glasses. Yes, she was four feet tall. But for me, an average-size person who assimilates into my consciousness the way dwarfs look every day of my life, the only thing that stood out about her appearance was that she pulled a hand cart with a stool and a pillow everywhere she went, the better with which to make herself comfortable following back surgery. As with Becky, it wasn't her height that I noticed so much as the complications of achondroplasia. The idea that anyone would scream because of her size was incomprehensible. Will people ever look at Becky and become so overwhelmed with fear and revulsion that the only thing they can do is scream?

With his training in psychology, Len Sawisch offers specific answers to the question *What is it about dwarfs?* He points to three reasons why dwarfs receive an inordinate amount of attention, even compared to people with other visible disabilities.

First, of course, they simply look different. "Our attention is drawn to incongruity," Sawisch explains. "Our attention is drawn to dissonance. Our attention is drawn to differentness. There is so much sensory stimulation available to us that we can't afford to tend to all of it, or most of it. So what we do is filter out the sameness." Dwarfs, obviously, do not get filtered out.

Second, we associate size with age, and dwarfs break that particular mold. "Everybody was once small, regardless of where you are as a human," Sawisch says. "We all grow at least some, and everybody went through that whole growth process or maturation process." And one of the lessons that kids learn, he adds, involves "size and power and freedom and autonomy and the ability to force your will on others." The message that kids hear is, "You're not big enough, you're not old enough. When you get older, when you get bigger, older/bigger, older/bigger." Dwarfism turns this simple childhood rule on its head.

Finally, there is the matter of "innate releasers," sensory stimuli that trigger the most instinctive, primitive parts of our brains to react in preprogrammed ways. Sawisch cautions that this is theory rather than established fact. But the idea is that dwarfs have certain characteristics that make people think of infants, and thus simply seeing them can conjure up some of the same emotions. Sawisch specifically cites achondroplastic dwarfs, whose large heads and small limbs mimic the proportions of babies. But the innate-releaser theory, if true, would presumably apply to other types of dwarfs as well.

Including Charles Stratton and Lavinia Warren. Unlike achondroplastic dwarfs, they had the same proportions as average-size adults, even though they were less than three feet tall. Yet surely the innate-releaser theory would apply to them, since their childlike appearance was their principal attraction. It was an attraction they were able to exploit their entire lives, for richer and poorer, in sickness and in health. At a time when the display of "human curiosities" was an ingrained part of American culture, General and Mrs. Tom Thumb figuratively stood above them all.

Charles and Lavinia Stratton's hold on the imagination persists. The Tom Thumb memorabilia is the highlight of the Barnum Museum in Charles's hometown of Bridgeport. Among other things, you can see several of the miniature carriages that the Strattons used, including one shaped like a walnut. On the wall opposite is an inscription that manages both to capture Tom Thumb's appeal and to strip Charles Stratton of his humanity: "Like a living Peter Pan, Tom Thumb seemed to bridge the gap between man and boy — to be a clever child who refused to grow up. People came to see him out of curiosity, but quickly identified with his spirit of mischief and fun."

It is in Middleborough, though, where the allure remains strongest. At the Tom Thumb Museum I picked up a sheet of paper with the outline of a tiny hand that is supposed to be that of "Mrs. Tom Thumb." The instructions: "Please place your hand on the drawing to get a better idea of her size." I also bought a book called *General Tom Thumb and His Lady* that turned out to be little more than a deification of its subjects, complete with endless descriptions of the gifts they received and their "fairy wedding."

I wondered whether I would ever take Becky to such a place. I liked Mrs. Beals, and the memorabilia was displayed with both affection and respect. Yet the prevailing atmosphere was that of a different, crueler era, a time when viewing "wonders of nature" such as the Strattons was seen as no more perverse than, say, keeping people as slaves. At the very least, I knew I didn't want Becky to see this until she was old enough to understand it fully. Surely it would never mean the same thing to her that it did to me when I was a child — that is to say, nothing much, just a place to while away a rainy afternoon.

After taking my leave of the museum, I stopped by the Middleborough Public Library. In one of the library's reading rooms, exactly as I remembered them, were enormous portraits of Charles and Lavinia; in another, Minnie Warren and Commodore Nutt.

But there was one more stop I wanted to make. I recalled that the Bump family lot was not twenty feet from where my parents were buried, in Nemasket Hill Cemetery. I drove up and started looking around. I found a weather-beaten old tombstone, a cross, a crown, and the name MINNIE inscribed on one side. On the other was a more complete description:

HULDAH P.
WIFE OF
EDWARD NEWELL
DAU. OF
J. S. & H. P. BUMP
BORN JUNE 2, 1849
DIED JULY 23, 1878

This was Minnie Warren, Lavinia's only dwarf sibling in a large family of large people. Minnie had become pregnant and, according to Mrs. Beals, was advised to have an abortion; but she rejected the idea on religious grounds. Sadly, because of her small size, both she and her child died. The baby was supposedly buried in its mother's arms, although there was no mention of that on the headstone. Her husband, also a dwarf, returned to his native England and remarried, later performing off and on with Lavinia and the Count.

Minnie's grave had one other noteworthy quality: rectangular stonework, covered with lichens, that outlined what must have been the dimensions of her child-size coffin.

Thus even in death was Minnie Warren singled out for her dwarfism. As with the figure of Seneb, benignly looking out over the expanse of more than four thousand years, balancing himself on stunted legs, his tiny arms held in front of him, Minnie's survivors made sure that her difference would transcend life itself. It says something interesting and maybe a little unsettling about us. Yes, she was a dwarf, but she was also a person — a person with dwarfism, if you will. To the living, though, it seems that her size was her most important characteristic.

Chapter Four

The Valley of the Shadow of Death

When Becky came home from Mass General, it was to a room that had been utterly transformed to cater to her new, intimidating needs. Rather than the small upstairs bedroom that we'd set aside for her, we rearranged what had been a large guest room on the first floor. A metal shelving unit held an oximeter, a wire from which we would attach to one of her big toes whenever she was sleeping; if the ideal oxygen level in her blood fell below 95 percent, an alarm would go off, and we would rush in to see what the problem was. If it fell below 90, it was time to think about getting her to the hospital. There was a suction machine to remove mucus and phlegm from her trach tube, a procedure we had to perform dozens of times a day. A basket filled with little plastic containers of saline solution, which helped to loosen the mucus. Extra trach ties. An enormous humidifier that delivered heated mist to her trach opening. A big green oxygen tank for home and a little portable oxygen tank for road trips.

And there were people, lots of them. Home nurses, wonderful women who were with us for as much as eighteen hours a day at first, tending to Becky while we slept, showing us the nuances of how best to meet her needs when we were awake. Technicians from a medical-supply company, miserable human beings who seemed not to know or care what they were doing. Occupational and physical therapists, well-meaning people who'd let their narrow areas of expertise somehow transmogrify into a condescending, we-know-best attitude that left us perplexed and infuriated.

What was most important about all of this, though, was that Becky herself was taken seriously. When she was first diagnosed with achondroplasia, the message was consistent: *She'll be fine.* During her two months in Mass General, we were told: *She'll be fine, once she gets through this.* And after she came home, it was: *She'll be fine, you just need to be patient.* A generation or two ago, the parents of a child just diagnosed with dwarfism were sometimes told that their baby might not live long (true enough in some cases), or could be mentally retarded, or might even be better off in an institution. By contrast, everyone we dealt with, even the ones we didn't like, took Becky's difference as a given, and treated her dwarfism not as a problem unto itself, but rather as a complication that made it difficult for her to breathe, or pick up a stuffed animal, or roll over, or sit up. Get her through all that, and yes, *She'll be fine.*

It's an attitude that's made all the difference in her life. And it's an attitude that would be inconceivable were we not a society that accepted difference — if not perfectly, if not in all cases, then at least to a far greater extent than we did a hundred years ago, when freak shows were giving way to science, and science, all too often, abandoned the pursuit of truth in favor of crackpot theories about genetic superiority that reflected nothing so much as the prejudices of those who espoused those theories. In the 1930s and 1940s these theories reached their logical, and terrible, conclusion in Nazi Germany, where conformity was held up as the highest ideal and difference was seen as something to fear, and to eliminate.

In a very real sense, the disability consciousness that came into being in the second half of the twentieth century, and which has done so much to enhance Becky's life and improve her prospects, sprang from the ashes of death camps such as Auschwitz and Dachau, where millions of innocent people met their fate. And at a little-remembered camp called Mauthausen, where one man's life and death symbolizes the horrifying consequences of regarding human difference as pathology.

He looks at the camera straight on. He is dressed in the striped prison garb of the Mauthausen concentration camp, in Austria. His face — grim but dignified, almost serene — betrays a terrible awareness. He knew what was coming next.

Sixty years ago Alexander Katan stared into the lens of a Nazi photographer's camera. Today he stares into the eyes of anyone who visits a website that documents his final moments. Move the cursor on top of his picture and it's replaced by something else: a skeleton, obviously that of a dwarf with limb deformities, propped up like a curiosity in a display case. It is the skeleton of Alexander Katan.

After poking around the Internet and gleaning a few details about Katan's life and death, I wrote to the Mauthausen Memorial Archives, hoping to learn more. In response, I received a letter from Dr. Doris Wagner, an official with Austria's Federal Ministry of the Interior. Katan, she wrote, was born in Rotterdam on November 18, 1899. After Germany overran the Netherlands, Katan was registered as a "Dutch Jew" (*Jude NL*). He was arrested and brought to Mauthausen on or about November 3, 1942. On January 27, 1943, camp officials ordered him killed with an injection to the heart — the better to preserve his remains — so that his skeleton could be displayed and photographed. Wagner did not say how the flesh was so neatly stripped from Katan's bones, leaving behind nothing but a perfect skeleton. But mostly likely his dead body was dipped in a vat of caustic chemicals.

Wagner's letter included images of some actual records pertaining to Katan's imprisonment and death. The cause of death was described as *Eitriger Dickdarmkatarrh*, or ulcerative colitis. Wagner's letter noted with clinical dispassion that "the given cause of death does not necessarily correlate with the actual reasons for the prisoner's demise."

Katan was not taken to Mauthausen because he was a dwarf, but because he was a Jew. Nor was he killed because he was a dwarf. The complex of camps that comprised Mauthausen, though not as well-remembered today as Auschwitz or Dachau, was a place of unimaginable cruelty, and only a small fragment of what went on was aimed at those who were physically different. An estimated 150,000 people were killed. Some were ordered to remove their clothes in subzero temperatures and then sprayed with water, freezing them to death. Some were hacked to pieces by pick-wielding sadists. Some were simply starved, left lying in pools of excrement until they stopped moving and, finally, stopped breathing.

But though Alexander Katan was imprisoned and killed because he was a Jew, the particular way in which he was killed — and the way his remains were displayed, ogled at, desecrated — had everything to do with the fact that he was a dwarf. The Nazis were obsessed with physical differences, seeing them as signs of weakness, of genetic impurities that needed to be stamped out. Such differences in a Jew were evidence — confirmation — of Nazi ideology, which held that Jews were racially inferior to the blond-haired, blue-eyed "Aryans" who were held up as the ideal of pure Germanic blood.

Perhaps Katan was killed on the orders of Dr. Eduard Krebsbach, who was reportedly the first Mauthausen physician to use heart injections to execute inmates whom he considered sick or otherwise unfit. Krebsbach's notoriety was such that he was nicknamed "Dr. Spritzbach" — that is, "Dr. Injection." His tenure at Mauthausen was cut short after he was caught shooting a hard-partying

German soldier on holiday who, along with his friends, had disturbed the good doctor's rest. But Dr. Injection and his fellow physicians left behind quite a legacy: 286 specimens of human organs, a collection that the camp assembled in collaboration with the SS Medical Academy, at the University of Graz. According to one account, the collection included "hearts, lungs, kidneys, faces, skeletons, and skulls" of inmates, murdered by heart injection "to preserve their anatomical 'anomalies.'" The attractions also included an album of tattooed skin, as well as lampshades and furniture made out of human remains.

The story of Alexander Katan, in many respects, traces our cultural attitudes toward difference in the first half of the twentieth century. Gradually, disability's place in social consciousness moved from the freak show to the laboratory, and not always for the good of the disabled. Under the guise of the then-new pseudoscience of eugenics, physical differences such as blindness, deafness, mental retardation (or "imbecility," as it used to be known), and the like were seen as something to study, to classify, to categorize. And to eliminate.

Dwarfism — as it had always been, as it is today — was seen as somehow different from other disabilities. There is no record of dwarfs having been specifically targeted by the eugenicists. Nor is there any evidence that dwarfs who were both healthy and mobile were considered disabled, not even by the Nazis. Yet as Katan's fate shows, dwarfs were not put in quite the same category as the able-bodied, either. Left alone in normal times, they were singled out for their difference during moments of social breakdown and cultural madness. Some, like Katan, suffered a fate worse than that of their average-size peers — worse not because he was killed (after all, he was hardly alone in that), but because of the way he was mocked even after his death. Some were allowed to live because they were different — as was the case with the Ovitzes, whom I will discuss later in this chapter, a family of Jewish dwarfs who survived Auschwitz only because the infamous Josef Mengele saved them for his experiments.

The identity politics that has come to define the disability community in recent decades is, in a sense, a direct, ongoing response to the eugenics movement, and to the ugly end to which it came in the 1940s. They include the deaf activists who label cochlear implants "genocide"; the wheelchair-users who rail against Christopher Reeve for seeking a cure for his quadriplegia rather than raising political consciousness; and the parents who changed the term *mongoloidism* to *Down's syndrome* and then later insisted that the possessive be dropped, lest it appear that those with the of the condition somehow were the property of the physician, Dr. J. Langdon Down, who first described it. Identity politics has also had an effect on the organized dwarf community, which at first rejected the disability label and then later embraced it as a way to advance its agenda of acceptance and access.

The overarching message voiced by all these activists is that disability is a difference, not a defect, and that difference is to be celebrated. From a purely scientific point of view, their logic is dubious. As Becky's pulmonary specialist, Dr. Dan Shannon, once told me, it makes no more sense to place a positive value on dwarfism than on diabetes. Is someone whose pancreas can't produce enough insulin an example of the rich tapestry of human diversity, or would her life instead be enhanced by the elimination of such diversity — that is, by a cure? The answer is obvious.

But illogical though the diversity model of disability may be, it has enormous worth in terms of politics and culture. Treating disability as though it were like race, sexual orientation, or religion — as something to be tolerated, accepted, protected, even celebrated — helps make this a more dignified, open, and just society. Treating it as a defect to be stamped out is divisive and deadening. At its worst, it leads to a display case in Mauthausen, where Nazi officials and doctors — members of the most thoroughly Nazified of all the German professions — peered thoughtfully at the skeleton of a deformed little man, the flesh stripped from his bones in just the right way so as not to interfere with their edification and amusement.

Eugenics was the bastard child of evolution and genetics. Charles Darwin's *Origin of Species*, published in 1859, introduced such ideas as natural selection and the survival of the fittest. The development of living things was removed from the realm of theology and transferred to that of science. Humans were not made in God's image — not directly, anyway — but, rather, evolved from ape-like ancestors millions of years ago, becoming more intelligent over time because intelligence gives humans an advantage over their competitors: predatory animals; the elements; and, most provocatively, less intelligent, and therefore less evolved, fellow humans.

Most scientists today believe that evolution is quite a bit more complicated and random than the onward-and-upward path described by Darwin, which bespoke a faith in progress every bit as theological, in its way, as the story of the Garden of Eden. In its time, though, Darwin's theory of evolution had an explosive effect. The notion that humans are evolving into an ever more intelligent and powerful species was as dangerous as it was exhilarating.

A cruel political philosophy known as Social Darwinism became popular in the latter half of the nineteenth century. Its adherents believed that the poor were responsible for their plight, and that they were somehow inferior, from an evolutionary point of view, to those who were more successful. Worse, Social Darwinists believed that society should refrain from helping the poor, because all they would do is reproduce and drag humanity down the evolutionary ladder with them. Those whites who had never accepted blacks as fully human now claimed to have additional evidence, arguing that blacks had not risen as far from apehood as whites had. In pop culture, to cite just one example,

P. T. Barnum exploited the public's hazy understanding of

evolution by displaying a microcephalic black man named William Henry "Zip" Johnson, whom he billed as "What Is It?" and described as the missing link between humans and orangutans.

Eugenics was the scientific — or, rather, pseudoscientific — counterpart to Social Darwinism. Fittingly enough, it was first promulgated by a cousin of Darwin's, Sir Francis Galton, who came up with the word and defined its purpose: to encourage those humans who were supposedly more evolved to reproduce as much as possible, and to discourage the lower sorts from breeding at all. His ideas about superiority matched up conveniently with his own ethnicity and social class. Though Galton was gifted enough as a scientist to develop the modern method of fingerprint identification, he could also be so sloppy and prejudiced that he actually sought to support his eugenics theory with data showing that successful people tend to be related to other successful people, as though that were the result of anything other than environment. (Then again, it's not as though those ideas have gone away entirely. Witness those who argue that the poor performance of black children on standardized tests is evidence of intellectual inferiority rather than differences in family history and opportunity or a cultural bias in the tests themselves.)

Darwin's theory of evolution was a necessary but not wholly sufficient basis for eugenics. The other element was genetics — the discoveries of Gregor Mendel, the obscure Austrian monk whose experiments with peas showed how inherited characteristics were handed down from one generation to the next. Eugenics, then, was a toxic combination of Darwin's theory of the survival of the fittest and Mendel's ideas about the mechanics of heredity. As Simon Mawer writes in his fine, quirky 1998 novel, *Mendel's Dwarf*, "It was a science that would ultimately lead to the ovens of Auschwitz."

Though eugenics reached its apex in Nazi Germany, it found a receptive home early on in the United States. Perhaps this is not surprising, given our belief in science and progress and self-improvement. Gradually, public display of the disabled came to be seen as barbaric. As Howard University's Rosemarie Garland Thomson writes, "Looking at disability became inappropriate in the same way that public executions and torture came to be considered offensive by the nineteenth century." It was around this time, Thomson observes, that the bleeding figure of Jesus began to disappear from the Protestant cross, a change that was emblematic of the "banishment of the image of disability." The medicalization of disability, she adds, led to another, even more disturbing shift in cultural attitudes: rather than being viewed as "natural wonders," the disabled came to be seen as something that was broken and therefore had to be fixed. Or cast aside. "The logic of 'cure or kill,' accompanied by today's faith in technology," writes Thomson, "posits that if the disabled body cannot be normalized, it must be eliminated."

Among the earliest, and weirdest, proponents of such elimination was Dr. Harry Haiselden, a young surgeon from Chicago who burst on the scene in 1915 when he told the *Chicago American*, a mass-market Hearst newspaper, that he had let a disabled newborn baby die. Like a proto-Jack Kevorkian, Haiselden was investigated three times for refusing to save the lives of disabled infants. Unlike Kevorkian, he evaded official censure. Ultimately, though, he was kicked out of the Chicago Medical Society for espousing his views in newspaper articles and for making a bizarre and disturbing movie called *The Black Stork*. Its message was not subtle. The mother of a disabled newborn must decide whether to let a surgeon save her baby, or to let him die. She has a vision: her surgically repaired child grows up to become a criminal who has disabled kids of his own. Ultimately, he tracks down the doctor who saved his life and kills him. Mom makes what was, from Haiselden's point of view, the right choice. As the film moves toward its conclusion, a faint image of Jesus is superimposed in the background, and the child's soul leaps into his waiting arms.

In the early part of the twentieth century, the United States led the world in putting eugenics theory into practice. It has been estimated that more than thirty thousand people were systematically sterilized in twenty-nine states — about half of them in California — between 1907 and 1939. These sterilizations were aimed primarily at mentally retarded or mentally ill people living in institutions and prisons, sometimes without their knowledge, sometimes against their will.

A particularly notorious case involved an eighteen-year-old woman named Carrie Bruck, who was living in an institution for the "feebleminded" in Virginia. As described by the disability historian Joseph Shapiro, Bruck was the middle actor in a multigenerational tragedy: she had just given birth, and her mother was warehoused in the same institution. It's likely that their real disability was poverty rather than any sort of mental deficiency, according to Shapiro. Nevertheless, state officials sought forcibly to sterilize Carrie Bruck, and the United States Supreme Court agreed. Wrote Justice Oliver Wendell Holmes Jr. in the 1927 opinion: "It is better for all the world, if instead of waiting to execute degenerate offspring for crime, or to let them starve for their imbecility, society can prevent those who are manifestly unfit from continuing their kind. . . . Three generations of imbeciles are enough!"

By comparison, Germany had a lot of catching up to do — so much so, according to the historian Robert Jay Lifton, that a German geneticist named Fritz Lenz complained in 1923 that Germany was lagging well behind the United States in sterilizing its undesirables. The Weimar constitution, Lenz noted with disdain, forbade alterations to the human body, a category that included vasectomies. Worse, he complained, the country had no laws to prohibit people with disabilities such as mental retardation or epilepsy from getting married. That would soon change — and Lenz himself would become a top official in Nazi Germany's eugenics programs.

It did not take long for Germany to assume a leadership position. Lifton makes an important point about the difference between the United States and Britain (another leading center of enthusiasm for eugenics) on the one hand and Germany on the other. The United States and Britain, with their open political systems and ingrained respect for individual rights, had self-correcting mechanisms in place that held the eugenic impulse at least somewhat in check. In Germany, where the Nazis quickly established a totalitarian state after rising to power in 1933, eugenics was imposed forcibly from above. Hitler himself once said that the state "must see to it that only the healthy beget children. . . . It must declare unfit for propagation all who are in any way visibly sick or who have inherited a disease and can therefore pass it on." His deputy, Rudolf Hess, put it more simply: "National Socialism is nothing but applied biology."

This applied biology took the form of two programs: mass sterilizations, which began in 1934, and direct killing — "euthanasia," as it was euphemistically called — which began in 1939. Using these means the Germans eliminated what they called *lebensunwerten Leben* — "life unworthy of life." The "euthanasia" program, in particular, was a dress rehearsal for the Final Solution. As the physician-murderers refined their techniques, they eventually hit upon an efficient system for doing away with the institutionalized disabled who were supposedly under their care: they would kill them with gas, then burn their bodies in a crematorium. The so-called euthanasia program was supposed to be kept a secret, but German opinion became inflamed as fact and rumor began to spread. In 1941 Hitler officially ended it, although it continued surreptitiously until the end of the war. The killing technology — the gas equipment and the ovens — were simply packed up and shipped to the death camps, where six million Jews and millions of others met their fates.

Overall, it has been estimated that between 300,000 and 400,000 people were sterilized during the Nazi era, and perhaps as many as

200,000 to 250,000 were killed under the various "euthanasia" programs.

But as terrible as these crimes were, it appears that dwarfs were largely spared. Sterilization and "euthanasia" were aimed almost exclusively at severely disabled people living in institutions. Above all, the Nazis were obsessed with mental conditions. Schizophrenia, epilepsy, manic-depressive illness, mental retardation, and the like accounted for well over half the cases of those who were murdered. Dwarfism was not mentioned in the list of physical conditions that the Nazis sought to eliminate, such as hereditary blindness or deafness. Certainly some severely disabled dwarfs already living in institutions may have been killed, since they would have been considered "life unworthy of life." But there is no evidence that healthy German dwarfs, living and working alongside their average-size fellow citizens, were singled out in any systematic way for sterilization or death. Still, there may have been exceptions.

The disability historian Hugh Gregory Gallagher has written in considerable detail about precisely which mental and physical disabilities the Nazis targeted for elimination, and although the list does not include dwarfism, he mentions dwarfs' being killed almost in passing. When I contacted Gallagher, he told me he had no specific documentation. But that doesn't mean that *no* dwarfs were targeted. Gallagher writes that, at its worst, "euthanasia" was meted out to anyone who didn't conform — a category far-reaching enough to encompass children in orphanages who had bad skin. Or bad attitudes. It seems possible that some dwarfs were victimized during this time simply because of their dwarfism, perhaps under the guise that they had severe hereditary physical disabilities, a catchall category that the Nazis also made use of. What really happened, though, remains a mystery.

One afternoon I paid a visit to the United States Holocaust Memorial Museum, in Washington, D.C., to interview Patricia Heberer, a historian of the Nazi war against the disabled. I was accompanied by Cara Egan, a woman with achondroplasia who has studied the role of the dwarf community in the disability-rights movement. "There's no consistent targeting of dwarfs or little people for the 'euthanasia' program,'" Heberer told us. "'Euthanasia' doesn't go beyond the bounds of the custodial setting. What they're doing is getting rid of a population in an institutional setting, and they're not concerned with people who can function, or who are outside that."

Afterwards, Andy Hollinger, a museum official, took Egan and me to an exhibit on the fate of the disabled under the Nazis. We saw a miserable little bed, body restraints, a physician's smock. Behind all this was an enormous photo of the crematory smokestack at the Hadamar mental institution, belching out the ashes of human remains — the setting for a surreal celebration of speechmaking and beer-drinking, vividly described by Hugh Gallagher, upon the occasion of the ten thousandth victim's death. There were photos, too, of mentally retarded children just before they were killed, of buses with the windows painted over so that no one could see in or out, of a doctor examining the body of a child who'd been "euthanized," supposedly so that he could study the genetic basis of disease.

Particulars are important. It's worth knowing whether dwarfs were or were not singled out by the Nazis. But it's even more important not to lose sight of the overarching horror of what took place.

Liebe Perla ("Dear Perla"), a 1999 film by the Israeli documentarian Shahar Rozen, is deceptively low-key. Its subject is a ten-member family of Hungarian-Jewish entertainers — seven of them dwarfs — who survived Auschwitz because of Josef Mengele's perverted curiosity. One of the survivors, an elderly dwarf named Perla Ovitz, is interviewed in her Haifa home by a German researcher, Hannelore Witkofski, who is herself disabled. Near the beginning of the film, Ovitz makes what the narrator calls "an unusual request." During their time in Auschwitz, Mengele had ordered the entire Ovitz family to be photographed naked. Perla Ovitz asks Witkofski to find the photo and bring it to her so that it can't be viewed by anyone else.

We follow Witkofski as she tries to track the photo down, in German archives and at the Auschwitz memorial. Apparently it is lost forever. What we do see, though, is profoundly chilling.

At one point we see a film clip of Jews being herded into Auschwitz, a dwarf clearly visible. At another, Perla receives word from Yad Vashem, the Holocaust memorial in Jerusalem, that her family's musical instruments have been found; she and Witkofsky make an emotional trip to see, to touch, the instruments upon the latter's return to Israel. Then there is Perla's ambivalence about Mengele — an ambivalence that is shocking given the evil he did to her family and to countless thousands of others. She recalls Mengele's eyeing the seven dwarfs when they arrived at Auschwitz and saying gleefully, "I've got work for twenty years." She remembers thinking: "God, I don't want to live twenty years." Yet she could not let go of the notion that it was Mengele who had saved them, that it was his interest in their dwarfism that allowed them to live. She tells Witkofski that she cried when she learned Mengele had died in Uruguay. "I can't say anything bad about him," she says. We see her nephews arguing with her, telling her it is unimaginable that she could hold such views about a monster such as Mengele.

In an interview with the journalist Yehuda Koren published after the film was released, Ovitz offered more details. She said that shortly after arriving at Auschwitz, her family was actually dragged off to the gas chambers against Mengele's orders. He rescued them, giving them milk so they would vomit out the poison that had already entered their bodies. They were poked and prodded, injected and inspected; Mengele took blood, marrow, teeth from them, but he never took their lives. "We were the only family who entered a death camp and emerged together," she told Koren. "If ever I questioned why I was born a dwarf, my answer must be that my handicap, my deformity, was God's way of keeping me alive." Mengele, she recalled, even made up a rhyme that he would chant: "Over the hills and seven mountains, there my seven dwarfs do dwell." After the war ended, they performed in Israel as the "Seven Dwarfs of Auschwitz."

For some in the dwarf community, it is an article of faith that the Nazis sought to eliminate all dwarfs. As Rika Esser, an official with *BundesselbsthilfeVerband Kleinwüchsiger Menschen*, the German little people's association, said to me in an e-mail, "I read quite a number of books on the Third Reich in general, and the fate of short people was only mentioned as a footnote, if ever. But: since the goal of the regime was to keep the 'German genes' as much Aryan (TALL, blond, blue-eyed) as possible, and since this is not reconcilable with being short, I guess that this in itself is a reason to prosecute dwarfs." Indeed, after I saw *Liebe Perla* at a screening with a couple of dozen Little People of America members, there was a heated discussion about that very topic. One person went so far as to say that, after World War II, there were few dwarfs left in Europe because Hitler had killed nearly all of them. There is no evidence of that — not in Robert Jay Lifton's or Hugh Gregory Gallagher's books, and not in any of the voluminous records that the Nazis kept about their evil deeds. Patricia Heberer, the Holocaust Museum historian, told Cara Egan and me that the dwarfs who were sent to the death camps were Jews, or perhaps members of some other persecuted group, mainly the Roma, better known as Gypsies.

In fact, *Liebe Perla* underscores the uniquely Jewish character of the Holocaust. Perla Ovitz told Koren that she and her family were able to continue touring and performing for several years during the war because they had hidden the fact that they were Jews. After Germany invaded Hungary, she recalled, "the Nazis gave us a hand, lifted us onto the packed train, and helped us find some space." Only later, when the authorities learned that the Ovitzes were Jews, were they sent to Auschwitz. Alexander Katan's papers identified him as a "Dutch Jew," and made no mention of his dwarfism. The same was presumably true of Lya Graf, a Jewish dwarf who performed in American circuses in the 1920s and 1930s and who became briefly famous when she was photographed sitting in the lap of the financier J. P. Morgan. Graf and her parents returned to their native Germany in the 1930s, and she died, along with her parents, at Auschwitz in 1941.

In her 1985 memoir of her time in Auschwitz, Sara Nomberg-Przytyk tells a story about a family of dwarfs that is almost unbearable to read. It is about another family of Hungarian-Jewish entertainers, circus performers in this case, comprising three dwarf women, two average-size women married to dwarfs, and a three-year-old boy who was the son of a dwarf but who was apparently average-size himself. The family members slobber all over Mengele, thanking him for saving them, but he will have none of it. Instead, he is inflamed with demented curiosity over their sex lives, particularly between the average-size women and the dwarf men. "You will tell me if the little one is the midget's son, or did you have him with somebody else?" he leers. Later, he takes the three-year-old and dissects him, while still alive. "Without blinking an eye," Nomberg-Przytyk writes, "Mengele was inflicting physical agonies on a three-year-old child who had not the least understanding of what was happening." The boy died that night.

So much has been written and said about Mengele that it is hard to know what more can be added. In reading about his life and career, two things struck me in particular. The first was his basic lack of intelligence. Mengele is often portrayed as some sort of evil genius, as in Gregory Peck's depiction in the 1978 film *The Boys from Brazil.* But as Gerald Posner and John Ware make clear in their biography of Mengele, the Angel of Death was really a hardworking B-student type who had convinced himself that his sadistic and worthless experiments — especially on twins, but to a lesser extent on dwarfs and others — would win him a university professorship after the war.

The other aspect of Mengele's personality worth noting was his simultaneous kindness and cruelty toward his victims, a quality that is sometimes cited as evidence of deep psychological problems. He may well have had such problems, but it seems more plausible to me that he was just evil. Having already thoroughly dehumanized his subjects, he simply thought of them as laboratory mice. A good scientist will keep his mice warm and well-fed, and maybe even murmur sweet nothings into their little ears from time to time. But that's not going to stop him from poking their eyes out, injecting them with poisons, and cutting them open when they're still alive so that he can see the effects of his experiments.

It is not entirely clear why Mengele was interested in dwarfs. Twins, yes: he wanted to learn the secret of multiple births so that he could help the German race multiply. But why dwarfs? It's thought that he saw dwarfism and other physical disabilities among Jews as evidence of racial inferiority, although that raises the question of what he made of Germans with the same conditions. He was also short himself, and on one occasion he reportedly drew a line on a wall in the children's block — at about the five-foot-two mark — with everyone under the line being sent to the gas chambers and those over it allowed to live another day. Was there a connection in his mind between his own mild short stature and the profound short stature of the dwarfs whom he tortured?

Within the dwarf community, one of the most celebrated books of recent years is Ursula Hegi's 1994 novel, *Stones from the River*. The lead character, Trudi Montag, is an achondroplastic dwarf — a *Zwerg* — whose life we follow from World War I until just after World War II, from childhood to early middle age. In literary terms, Trudi's dwarfism serves to make her a permanent outsider — a keen observer who is in, but never quite of, her time and place. Only once does her dwarfism put her at risk, even though other people with disabilities have disappeared from her village, never to be seen again. She is taken prisoner, and fears it is because the authorities have learned that she and her father have been hiding Jews in their basement. It turns out that she had been picked up because of an offhand remark she'd made, and, after three weeks, she is released — but not before this exchange with a Gestapo officer:

> He said: "The rules that used to temper curiosity no longer exist."
>
> She waited, confused.
>
> "Do you understand what I say?"
>
> "No."
>
> "You should. Don't you know what can happen to someone like you in our country?"
>
> *The Buttgereit boy . . . the man-who-touches-his-heart . . . the Heidenreich daughter* . . . No, she was not like them.
>
> "You become an experiment . . . a medical experiment for the almighty profession," he said, and told her of operations performed on twins, on people afflicted with otherness. "Because the rules that used to temper curiosity no longer exist . . . Some people might even tell you that a *Zwerg* has no right to live."
>
> She felt her back seize up on her. Bracing herself against the familiar heaviness at the base of her spine, she asked, "And you? Is that what you believe?"
>
> He looked at her, evenly, and she read in his eyes what she'd known four years before — that he didn't believe in anything or anyone.

In such a context it hardly matters that dwarfism was not among the differences that had been singled out as no longer being bound by "the rules that used to temper curiosity." It could be used as a threat. If today the deaf were at risk of being exterminated and dwarfs were not, well, what of tomorrow? And what would happen to someone like Trudi if she fell afoul of the authorities because of her opposition to the Nazis?

There were, after all, Germans who ended up at the death camps, too — political dissidents, gays and lesbians, and various and assorted misfits. If Trudi had been taken to Auschwitz for her political beliefs, forced to labor beneath the metal gate emblazoned with *Arbeit Macht Frei* ("Work Brings Freedom"), well, what would have happened to her then? Would she have fallen into Mengele's clutches? Would she have been killed under the 14f13 program, in which physicians who were veterans of the "euthanasia" movement were sent to the death camps to weed out those who were physically unable to perform their share of the work?

In the crematoria of Auschwitz and Mauthausen and the other death camps, millions died — and an ideology died as well. A half-century of trying to eliminate difference reached its logical, terrible conclusion. In the nineteenth century, the disabled were displayed as freaks of nature. In the first part of the twentieth, they were regarded as contaminants in the gene pool. Eugenics, finally, was exposed as the fraud and the evil that it was.

In 2000, the Dutch documentarian Hedda van Gennep made a film called *Dood Spoor?* ("Dead End?"), subtitled "A Son Seeks His Father." Van Gennep tells the story of Alphons Katan, Alexander Katan's son, and his successful quest to persuade officials at the Mauthausen Memorial to remove photographs of his father, several of which were taken after he had been stripped of his clothes. We learn some details of Alexander Katan's life — of his work as a tutor, of his strict observance of the Sabbath, of his and his wife's arrest and imprisonment. Alphons Katan's story is moving, even heartbreaking.

But I cannot agree with his crusade. We must bear moral witness, even when it's painful, even when it's intrusive, even when we might rather look away. Think of the haunted faces in those images from the killing fields of Cambodia, or of the piled-up bodies outside the churchyard in Rwanda. Avoiding the true nature of evil only increases the chance that it will happen again.

The photographs that were taken of Alexander Katan in his last moments are more than a document of one man. They are a message, a warning of what happens when we turn human variation into pathology, difference into defect — when we look at a person with a disability and see only the disability.

Alexander Katan belongs to the ages. He belongs to us, if we're capable of understanding what he's telling us.

Chapter Five

Chaos Theory

The first time I caught a glimpse of the spiritual was while I was recovering from the serious bout of depression that followed the deaths of my parents — my father in 1985, my mother in 1988. I couldn't define it, couldn't put my finger on it, couldn't even say when or where, never mind how. But it was real, and I stopped calling myself an agnostic.

The second time was in the spring of 1993, not long after Becky had come home from the hospital. Sometimes in the evening, Tim — "Timmy" then — would put a pillow in my lap while I was sitting on the floor, take a few steps back, and then make a running leap on top of me. Becky thought this was hysterical. Her eyes and mouth would open wide, her head would shake, her face would turn red, and out through her trach tube would come this nearly silent, breathy laugh.

After months of being an object, of having things done *to* her, she transformed herself before my eyes into a subject — a fully autonomous person, a little girl who, despite the trach tube, the oxygen tank, the suction machine, the nurses, and the piles of paperwork we had to deal with to keep all of that coming, had a mind of her own, and a very definite idea of what was funny. Her birth, and Tim's, had seemed miraculous, of course, but this was a rebirth — a rekindling of the promise that we'd seen those first few months and that had all but disappeared during those weeks in the hospital.

At a few minutes before ten-thirty on the morning of Sunday, April 11, 1993, we wormed our way into the back of the Northshore Unitarian Universalist Church and squeezed into the handful of remaining seats. Tim squirmed like a typical two-year-old. Becky was propped in her basket between Barbara and me, a clear plastic tube running from the mask over her trach to a portable oxygen tank on the floor, a metal-and-plastic contraption that was about the size of two large shoeboxes and that was transported by means of a shoulder strap.

Becky had been home for less than a week. There was a hint of spring in the air, and we were determined to resume as normal a life as possible. Like many parents of our generation, Barbara and I had been talking for some time about finding a church in which to raise our kids. Given our divergent religious views, the local Unitarian Universalist church seemed like a good place to try. For one thing, the Northshore church was just a couple of miles from our house. For another, we needed a place that was as spiritually broad-minded as possible.

Barbara was a Catholic, although by 1993 she was looking for something else. I was the son of a non-church-going Unitarian mother and an ex-Catholic, agnostic father. They had sent me to an Episcopal church for a few years in a less-than-successful attempt to make my grandmothers happy. (My maternal grandmother, who trotted off to the Unitarian church in Middleborough every Sunday, didn't care one way or the other. My paternal grandmother, on the other hand, was convinced that anything other than a Catholic upbringing would guarantee my eternal damnation.) Barbara and I had been married in a Catholic church by a priest and a Unitarian

Universalist minister — the last time, except for weddings and funerals, that either of us had stepped inside a house of worship. A confirmed agnostic during my teens and twenties, by this point I was looking for something else, too.

We were impressed by what we saw that morning. It was billed as an "Easter-Passover" service. As we were soon to learn, the church was home for a number of mixed Jewish-Christian couples, and since Unitarian Universalism espouses no particular creed, it was natural to pay homage to both. The highlight was an African folk tale acted out by the children of the church, which also spoke to something emblematic about UUs: we are overwhelmingly white, and liberal guilt over that fact is one of the denomination's defining characteristics. It so happens that the current president of the Unitarian Universalist Association, the Reverend William Sinkford, is African-American, but it remains a church influenced far more by Ralph Waldo Emerson and Henry David Thoreau than by either of the Reverends Martin Luther King.

One thing we did *not* do that day was stay until the end of the service. This was Becky's first trip away from the big oxygen tank at home, and every few minutes we looked anxiously at the gauge on the portable unit. Not long after eleven o'clock, we could see that the tank would soon be empty if we didn't get out of there. So we packed up our stuff, headed back to the car, and drove home. We later learned that the gauge on the tank was not working properly, and that there was more oxygen remaining than we'd thought. So we were able to return in the following weeks. We have been members ever since.

Because we live in a culture that encourages a view of God as someone who listens to our appeals and then decides whether to bestow favors upon us or torment us, the arrival of a child with a disability — any disability — can spark a crisis of faith. I have heard of people who literally ceased to believe in God because their child, or their grandchild, was diagnosed with dwarfism. Their reasoning: *A loving God would not do such a thing.* That's bad enough. Worse is when disability is viewed as a sign of divine disapproval.

I recall a conversation I once had with my mother when I was quite young. The teenage daughter of a neighbor had had a child out of wedlock, and the baby had some sort of disability. I can't recall what precisely the disability was, but it was something like a cleft palate or a clubfoot — in other words, a physical difference that would not cause overwhelming impairment but that was very visible. Apparently the neighbor had told my mother that *her* mother — in other words, the baby's great-grandmother — had said that the disability was God's punishment for the teenager's wanton sexuality. My mother was shocked that anyone could say something so hurtful and so hateful — and that this woman could actually believe that an innocent baby would be maimed by a vengeful God for the sole purpose of sending a message about the penalties of sin. Thus at an early age did my mother introduce me to two important concepts: that disability is just one of those things that sometimes happens, and that some people hold some exceedingly peculiar ideas.

This kind of thinking may not be as prevalent as it was a generation or two ago, but the notion that disability is a form of punishment persists. When Becky was born, Barbara wondered if she hadn't eaten enough of the right things, or had eaten too much of the wrong things; or if the treatments she'd taken to get pregnant and to reduce the chances of a miscarriage might have been the cause. I told her that feeling guilty was a waste of energy. We later learned that achondroplasia is tied to the *father*, especially to advanced paternal age; I was thirty-five when Becky was conceived, which, geneticists say, qualifies as advanced. And no, I didn't feel guilty.

Wondering about nutrition and fertility drugs and paternal age is a new twist on a very old theme. Throughout most of history, disability has been viewed as a sign of some sort of heavenly intelligence, evidence that God is trying to send us a message. All too often, it is seen as proof of moral failure — whether it's a failure to pray correctly, to live correctly, or, now, to eat correctly. It's a viewpoint that is not just wrong, but dangerous — dangerous to my daughter, dangerous to all of us. For it is one of the principal means by which we identify disabled people as the Other, as being somehow morally responsible for their differences, and are therefore defined by — and dismissed for — those differences.

This is not a mere theoretical or philosophical consideration, for it shapes how we interact with the disabled — whether we put them on display, treat them as objects of pity, organize our charitable efforts around them, or cut back on funding for their medical care during times of economic uncertainty. Our most deeply held beliefs about disability, rooted in religion or in such New Age offshoots as the cult of fitness, govern how we treat real people with real physical differences. As I write this, the Commonwealth of Massachusetts is making plans to eliminate health coverage for some fifty thousand adults who are what is euphemistically called the "long-term unemployed." You can be sure that people with some sort of disability are disproportionately represented in this group, whether it's mental illness, mobility problems (prosthetics are among the items that will no longer be available), or some other difference.

The state does face a genuine budget crisis. But at the root of these proposed cuts is the idea that buying artificial legs for poor people isn't something that we're obligated to do. Rather, it's something we do out of the goodness of our hearts, and we can't be expected to raise taxes on corporations or wealthy people so that we can keep on doing it in the midst of a recession.

This moral position would be unimaginable if it weren't for its unspoken, unconscious corollary: *It's their own fault.*

The idea that disability is a sign of God's disfavor can be traced back to the Bible, to at least Leviticus, in which God specifically forbids people with a wide range of physical deformities and maladies — including dwarfism — from serving as priests. The relevant passage in the King James version bans from the priesthood "a blind man, or a lame, or he that hath a flat nose, or any thing superfluous, or a man that is broken-footed, or broken-handed, or crookbacked, or a dwarf, or that hath a blemish in his eye, or be scurvy, or scabbed, or hath his stones broken." This prohibition helped establish a Judeo-Christian orientation toward disability that is ambiguous at best, hostile at worst. Subsequently, American and Western religious attitudes toward disability have been shaped primarily by Christianity. But as is so often the case with religion, it is left to us to decide which interpretation we wish to embrace. The liberal Protestant theologian Martin E. Marty lays claim to an enlightened Jesus, writing,

> I like the matter-of-factness of Jesus when they asked him about the man born blind; Jesus says, "Did he sin or did his parents, you ask me? He was born blind. Things just happen." *It rains on the just and the unjust alike.* [Marty's emphasis.]

But though it's comforting to think of Jesus as having a modern attitude toward the disabled, it's unlikely that an itinerant Jewish preacher who lived two thousand years ago actually would have held such views. And there is much evidence to the contrary. Take, for instance, this passage from John:

> As he walked along, he saw a man blind from birth. His disciples asked him, "Rabbi, who sinned, this man or his parents, that he was born blind?" Jesus answered, "Neither this man nor his parents sinned; he was born blind so that God's works might

be revealed in him."

Now, it's hard to know exactly what to make of this. The Reverend John W. Yates II, an Episcopal priest from Falls Church, Virginia, writes that Jesus is specifically rejecting the notion that the disabled are to blame for their condition. "He seems to be saying: 'Rather than looking backwards, let's look forward and ask what good thing might possibly come out of this,'" Yates writes. Yet Jesus also appears to be claiming some sort of special status for the disabled. Yates quotes from the New Revised Standard Version of the Bible; but in the New English Bible, whose editors claim is a more authoritative translation, Jesus answers his disciples that "he was born blind so that God's power might be displayed in curing him," a more explicitly utilitarian interpretation. Jesus spoke in metaphor and allegory and parable, and maybe this was the only way he could teach his followers that the disabled are not to be reviled. And of course, it's better to be exalted than damned, although either makes it difficult for a disabled person to lay claim to being fully human.

The disability historian Hugh Gregory Gallagher has a more malign interpretation of Jesus' ministry, writing, "Even the wise and gentle Jesus said to the blind man, 'I have healed you, go and sin no more,' implying, thereby, that sinning has brought on his blindness." Gallagher brings this frame of reference up to date by noting that gay people with AIDS are sometimes blamed for their illness because of their sexual activities, and that others with genuine maladies are dismissed by doctors who attribute their problems to psychosomatic causes. These are all variations on the same theme: *It's their fault.*

In our society, examples of John Yates's and Hugh Gallagher's interpretations are both easily found. That is, disabled people are either elevated as having special status or they are dismissed as having been singled out because of some innate shortcoming. In either case, the disabled person is an object, not a subject, someone who is acted upon rather than an actor in his or her own right. What we see all too rarely is the acceptance described by Martin Marty, taking the disabled as they are, fully human, with all of the strengths and weaknesses and hopes and desires and despair as anyone else.

One Columbus Day, we spent an afternoon at the Topsfield Fair, an annual event on Boston's North Shore featuring farm exhibits, games, and carnival rides. Near the end of an enjoyable day, I handed Becky a ticket so that she could take one more turn on a kiddie roller-coaster. I watched as she made several attempts to give her ticket to the grizzled old man who was operating the ride. He wouldn't take it, and I was afraid he was going to throw her off for not making the minimum height requirement, even though she'd been riding it all day without incident and even though I knew she was — just barely — tall enough. But he let her on, and she took several spins, laughing and waving as I waved back. She got off, still clutching her ticket. "I tried to give it to him," she told me. "It's all right," the man gruffly interjected. "I have a daughter who's handicapped."

What could I do, other than say "thank you" and move on? Fortunately the exchange seemed to elude Becky. But I was stunned. My daughter was getting charity at an amusement park merely because she was different-looking. And she was getting it from someone whose own life experience should have taught him that most disabled people would rather stand on their own two feet, whether they're able to do that literally or just figuratively. His use of the word "handicapped" was in itself interesting. Though the oft-told tale that it derives from a beggar's "cap in hand" appears to be a myth, the real etymology is no less significant. It comes from an old-fashioned game of chance known as "hand in cap," a game whose complex rules led to the modern meaning of *handicap*: to give an advantage to lesser competitors in games such as golf and horse-racing in order to level the playing field. Apparently my perfectly healthy, beautiful daughter could not enjoy a level playing field on that particular day without being given a free ride on a roller-coaster. She tried to act, making several attempts to give her ticket to the operator. Instead, she was acted upon.

Religion — or, rather, a specific way of thinking about religion — was at the root of what happened at the Topsfield Fair. It is an attitude that attained its full flowering in the nineteenth century. According to Peter Hall, a historian of philanthropy, Americans thought of the disabled as having been created by God so that others could practice their Christian virtues. Charles Dickens's sentimental *A Christmas Carol* was wildly popular in the United States of the 1840s, and its most popular character, Tiny Tim, was an object of pity. The disabled were seen as cut off from normal human desires — especially sexual urges — and to have almost a holy aura. "They have a purity about them which people feel they need to be connected to in some way," Hall told the documentarian Laurie Block, founder of the online Disability Museum, several years ago.

Block herself, who has a daughter with spina bifida, has talked about visiting the American Antiquarian Society in Worcester and finding "more than two hundred tales of moral instruction," written between the 1820s and the Civil War, about children with various disabilities, such as deafness and blindness. She recounts one story about a girl whose leg is to be amputated and who is lamenting her fate. (This was before anesthesia, mind you.) The voice that the girl hears in her head asks of her, "Is this the way you suffer the will of your Lord?" In the end, she pulls through with the support of her Sunday-school teacher. The message, Block says, is that children must be submissive and be willing to bear terrible pain. Once the child accepts that suffering, "he or she becomes worthy of God's grace and of charity."

Becky's experience with unsolicited charity notwithstanding, the tenuous relationship between disability in general and dwarfism in particular makes it hard to discuss its religious aspects in a way that is meaningful. Laurie Block didn't say so, but I seriously doubt that any of the two hundred children's tales she reviewed involved dwarfs. According to the Bible, Jesus made the blind see, the lame walk, and, in at least one instance, the dead spring back to life. But if he ever made a dwarf grow, there is no record of it. In an odd kind of way, Leviticus was millennia ahead of its time for categorizing dwarfism with other disabilities. For most of recorded history, the Tiny Tims of the world are worthy of our sentiment, but dwarfs are seen as wonders of nature, aberrations, freaks. Dwarfs are simultaneously part of and apart from disability culture, a duality that continues to this day.

But though people can argue over whether dwarfism is, in fact, a disability, there is no doubt that its complications can *cause* disabilities — and that those problems can change the way others view his place in the universe.

To gain some perspective, I spent a day with Susan and Curtis Forsley at their suburban home in Wells, Maine. Susan, who was forty-four at the time that I interviewed her, is a pleasant, intelligent woman of deep religious convictions. Curtis, nine, is a happy, active boy with achondroplasia who faces daunting challenges: he's already had brain-stem and spinal-decompression surgeries, and he also has Asperger syndrome, a type of autism that his mother believes may be related to the fact that his brain stem was being squeezed in utero and during his first months of life. Susan's husband and Curtis's father, Alex, is a merchant marine and was away at sea during my visit.

Curtis was still recovering from his most recent surgery, and Susan had to ask him continually to stop jumping around — an order that any nine-year-old would have a hard time with, never mind one who is locked into the repetitive behavior patterns of Asperger's.

Curtis's short stature has always been secondary to his medical needs. When he was four months old, doctors in Maine found that his foramen magnum was compressing his brain stem so tightly that he was on the verge of quadriplegia. He had a significant amount of hydrocephalus, too. He needed surgery immediately, the Forsleys were told — and, oh, by the way, they learned that their son was a dwarf as well.

"When we found out about the achondroplasia, it was a life-or-death situation, so all we cared about was our little baby being alive," Susan told me. "The dwarfism piece — as far as the social implications of that — we really haven't dealt with as much as we've dealt with the medical stuff. Now we have the autism piece. I think the autism piece is going to be harder to deal with than just the social dwarfism stuff. We're going from medical crisis to medical crisis, hoping to keep our baby alive and hoping to give him the best quality of life that he can have."

Asperger's is considered a high-functioning type of autism, and Curtis comes across as a smart kid. While his mother made us lunch, we watched television, and he explained the finer points of *SpongeBob SquarePants* to me. But some of his behavioral patterns are clearly inappropriate, and Susan wonders how independent he'll ever be. He flaps his arms. He has a hard time making eye contact. When he gets agitated he chews on electrical cords, or licks the floor or the kitchen counter. Once, she said, he even started licking another kid's hair during a church service.

Yet, if anything, these challenges have only deepened her religious faith. She told me that before she and Alex even knew each other, she worked for a time with Wendy Ricker — the mother of my friend Ruth Ricker — and thus knew where to turn after Curtis was diagnosed with dwarfism. "Divine intervention," she said. As for all of Curtis's various medical needs, and Alex's frequent absences, she told me that she never could survive if it weren't for the support provided by the Congregational church to which she belongs and which has come through with everything from meals to prayer groups.

I then asked her what I knew was a delicate question. *If you think it's wise to pray to help Curtis, why do you think God did this to him in the first place?* Her response: "I don't think he did this to him in the first place. I guess my belief — I've never questioned why, I never did. And the way I conceptualize it in my mind is that Curtis's soul was out there, waiting for somebody. And I feel chosen. I feel that God chose Alex and me as the best parents for Curtis. That, I guess, is my philosophical belief. That everybody has their cross to bear, everybody has something, everybody is a little different." She added, "There's a whole plan that we have no idea about, you know what I mean? A lot of people think, oh, you're too much of a Pollyanna. I've had a lot of parents say you're too sweetsie-sweetsie. But I've been there in real dark times, and I feel God's blessed us with this beautiful guy, and he's helped us. It is a challenge, but I wouldn't have it any other way. I really wouldn't."

Susan Forsley's religious beliefs are obviously heartfelt, and she voices them with real conviction. They are not wrong — for her. For me, though, it makes no more sense that an all-powerful God would seek out unusually good parents to care for disabled children than it does that an all-powerful God would inflict disabled children on sinful parents in order to punish them. These two beliefs are, in a sense, not terribly different from one another. Each starts from the same set of religious assumptions, but one takes a positive spin, one a negative.

Closely related to that is the aphorism that *God never burdens any of us with more than we can handle.* But this is obviously not true. I recently looked up an article that had made a deep impression on me years earlier. It appeared in the *New York Times* in 1995, and it related stories told by tens of thousands of refugees who were fleeing Bosnia in order to escape rampaging Serb forces. The refugees talked of mass rapes and murders, of entire families being killed. A woman who was about twenty years old made it to a refugee camp only to hang herself during the night. Another woman, eight months' pregnant, said, "People are beginning to go mad, especially the children who saw their fathers and brothers killed." If there is such a thing as an all-powerful, all-knowing God, clearly he burdened these people with more than they could handle. Stories such as these can be multiplied over and over, both on a macro scale (the Holocaust, Iraq, Rwanda) and on a micro scale (a child dies shortly after birth, a teenager is killed in a car accident, a family is wiped out in a house fire). Couples divorce. People go insane, or commit suicide.

I guess God works in mysterious ways.

If the idea that God would visit disabled children upon sinners is monstrous (and it is), or if the notion that he would choose special parents to raise disabled children is illogical (if he's *that* powerful, why did he create disabled children in the first place?), then are there any good, sound alternatives to consider?

Is there a genuine spirituality that does not assume the existence of an all-knowing, all-powerful God? Or is atheism, or its more intellectually respectable cousin, agnosticism, the only answer?

I asked the Reverend Paul Stevens Lynn, the pastor of Christ Lutheran Church in DuBois, Pennsylvania. Steve Lynn, who was forty-nine years old when we spoke, is an achondroplastic dwarf, one of the few little people in the United States — and, no doubt, the world — to serve as a member of the clergy. At four-foot-six, he is a foot shorter than his average-size wife, Lois Laine. According to Lynn, what's missing from the disability-as-punish-ment/disability-as-gift conundrum is the notion of free will. "God doesn't cause me to be a dwarf, or you to have had that accident and now to be a paraplegic, or your husband to have just died, or your child to commit suicide," he said. "Most of the time he *allows* those things to happen. Sometimes he intervenes, and that's called a miracle." He added, "God didn't cause me to be short. He allowed it to be. It's a difficult thing, but he didn't cause it. He loves me as I am, he's sorry for my pain, and he gets me through. He is a loving God, but he loves you so much that he doesn't control everything."

Well, what of the idea that God doesn't give people more than they can handle? "I would modify that," Lynn said. "God doesn't give anyone more than they can handle if they turn to him for help." *And what of the notion that Jesus said disability and sin are related, as Hugh Gallagher argues?* "Jesus was saying that it was much more important for a person to be forgiven sins than to be healed physically. They're not related," Lynn replied. "The real healing isn't the physical affliction. The real healing is the forgiveness of sins."

What Lynn is talking about, essentially, is the idea of God as love — God not as the cause of pain, but, rather, as the source of comfort during times of pain. This is similar to the God of Rabbi Harold Kushner's classic 1981 book, *When Bad Things Happen to Good People*, an extended modern-day meditation on the Book of Job. "I no longer hold God responsible for illnesses, accidents, and natural disasters, because I realize that I gain little and I lose so much when I blame God for those things," Kushner writes. "I can worship a God who hates suffering but cannot eliminate it, more easily than I can worship a God who chooses to make children suffer and die, for whatever exalted reason."

I read Rabbi Kushner's book after I received an e-mail from him and his wife, Suzette. I had made one of my semi-regular appearances as a media commentator for a local public-television show, *Greater Boston*, and the host, Emily Rooney, gave me several minutes to expound on my own book project. The Kushners happened to be watching that evening.

As everyone who has read *When Bad Things Happen* knows,

Kushner was prompted to write it because of the death of his son, Aaron, from progeria, a genetic condition that causes dramatically premature aging. What few people know is that the Kushners for a time took part in Little People of America events, short stature being one of the effects of progeria.

When Bad Things Happen to Good People is a wise and humane book. To Kushner, the disabled are subjects, not objects; actors, not pawns that have been acted upon by a God whose purposes we cannot comprehend. I am far more comfortable with that concept of God than with a supreme being who uses — abuses, for there is no other way to put it — his power by treating disability as a way to dispense punishment and favors. And yet I cannot fully accept this interpretation either.

God-talk does not come easily or naturally to me. It is far simpler to write about what I *don't* believe than what I do. Maybe it's because my one deeply held spiritual belief is that uncertainty is the only certainty, and that what's really important is to face the world with an open mind and an open heart, to be attuned to the possibility of things we don't understand. That's a hard rule to live by — I don't think I'm very good at living by it, actually — but, to me, it's the only rule that makes sense. I don't believe in an all-knowing, all-powerful God who directs our daily lives, but that doesn't make me an atheist or an agnostic, either. I don't rule out a divine intelligence — or, more likely, a divine love — that courses through the universe. The Reverend Forrest Church, the minister of the Unitarian Church of All Souls in New York City, could be speaking for me when he writes,

> The God I believe in now is different from the God I did not believe in when I was younger. . . . The God I believe in is neither male nor female nor any divine combination of the two. All this

I know, or think I know. On the other hand, I do not know, and never will know, just what the God I believe in is. The God I believe in will remain a mystery.

I believe that the universe is largely defined — as the minister of our church, the Reverend Ed Lynn, puts it — by "randomness and chaos." Far from being a bleak vision, I find this invigorating. Yes, it means things just happen. But it also means that each of us is in control of our own destiny, within whatever limitations we were born with or acquired along the way. Becky is not a dwarf because she deserves it, or because her parents are being punished, or because she or we have been chosen or singled out as somehow being special. Rather, she's a dwarf because of a random genetic mutation. She's got thirty thousand genes, and one is different from most people's. She is a subject, not an object. She is her own agent, the shaper of her own identity. Her disability is not her fault or our fault. It just *is*.

I don't think too many people would disagree with that, and yet, collectively, we act as though we are governed by the old superstitions. As I write this, the voters of Massachusetts have just rejected by a shockingly close margin — 55 percent to 45 percent — a proposal to do away with the state's income tax. If passed, it would have required that $9 billion be eliminated from the state budget, most of that, you can be sure, to come from social and medical services. When the tax cut's principal proponent, Carla Howell, a leading figure in the state's Libertarian Party, was asked how such drastic spending cuts would be offset, her answer was that people would boost their charitable contributions. But charity turns every person with a disability into Tiny Tim: an opportunity for others to convince themselves of how good and pious and worthy of heaven they are.

Once, toward the end of Becky's two years with a tracheostomy, I asked a social worker at our health-insurance company to help me figure out how much financial assistance we had received. It proved to be an impossible task, but in rough terms we came up with somewhere between a half and three-quarters of a million dollars. A lot of that was insurance money, especially for the weeks that she'd spent in the hospital. But a lot of it was public money, taxpayers' money, money that you and I and everyone else had sent to the government, grousing all the while about politicians and bureaucrats and waste and fraud and abuse.

In two years, we never received less than seventy-two hours of home nursing care a week, and such care is expensive. It was paid for by the Kaleigh Mulligan program, a state-federal partnership that covers home health services for children whose families make too much money to receive public assistance via the usual routes. The program was named for a real girl in Massachusetts who had Down syndrome and a variety of Down's-related ailments. And it saved our lives. Without it, Becky would have had to be placed in a chronic-care hospital, and we would have gone deep into debt. With it, not only could she live and grow and love and be loved at home, but the financial impact on us was minimal. The Kaleigh Mulligan program costs Massachusetts taxpayers about $8.5 million a year, less than it would take to put these children in hospitals. No, society can't pay for everything, and choices must be made. But is there really any doubt what is the right choice when it comes to the care of disabled children?

It could easily have been otherwise in a culture in which the disabled and their families are seen as being somehow responsible for their own misfortunes, as having offended God, or as having been sent to inspire acts of Christian charity. What was available to us — good health insurance and a compassionate government that filled in the gaps — should be available to everyone as a matter of right, not charity. What makes that possible is a mindset that regards genetic diversity as something good, and that sees all of us as part of the same human family.

Chapter Six

A Different Kind of Disability

Jacqueline Ann Clipsham is a formidable presence. She is a remarkably eclectic woman — a sculptor, a writer, a feminist, a veteran of the civil-rights movement, a disability activist, and a political radical whose bookcase is filled with back issues of *Marxist Perspectives.* But what sticks in my mind most is her surprising baritone voice, her authoritative demeanor, and her deeply held convictions about subjects ranging from race in America to the cruelties of the educational system in Britain, where she was born and spent part of her youth. I don't mean to encourage the idea that big is good, small is bad. But Jacki Clipsham is larger than life.

Clipsham, who has achondroplasia, was sixty-five years old when we met at her home in western New Jersey, near the Pennsylvania border. She rode her stairlift down to the front door to greet me. Clipsham lives in a big house back in the woods with plastic pink flamingoes out front. She is three-foot-ten, and gets around with the help of a walker, an electric scooter, and a specially modified van. There's a sculpting studio in the basement that's been modified right down to the kiln, which has a door on either side so that she doesn't have to do too much reaching. I ducked as she gave me a tour. "Some people have to stoop because the ceilings are too low," she said, watching me. "And I just say, 'Revenge!'"

I really hadn't known what to expect; I'd made an appointment with Clipsham because I'd been told she was an interesting person. She was certainly that. As it happened, she also turned out to be the ideal person to talk about the relationship between dwarfism and disability — a relationship that she figured out decades ago and that she complains has taken the dwarf community, and especially Little People of America, all this time to embrace. It's something that began forming in her mind when she was growing up in the Midwest and learned a life-altering lesson about people who are different.

"One of the interesting and important experiences I had was from the time I was in the second grade, old enough to walk to school, I would be called names, harassed, and made to feel threatened," she told me. "'Midget, midget,' all the usual garbage — mostly prepubescent boys, you know. At this point I noticed that the only other people who had a similar experience were black folks. They were harassed and called names and screamed and yelled at. Later on, I realized that when they got home, there were people like them. When I got home, there was nobody like me. And this was the seed of my political activism."

In 1964, Clipsham was a young sculptor working in Port Chester, New York, when three young civil-rights workers — James Chaney, Andrew Goodman, and Michael Schwerner — were killed in Philadelphia, Mississippi. Clipsham, who was already a member of the Congress on Racial Equality, or CORE, dropped what she was doing and volunteered at a community center in Sumter, South Carolina. She taught black children to appreciate African art, jazz, and blues — parts of their cultural heritage that they had been told was primitive and unworthy — and helped them overcome terrible nutritional deficiencies by cooking up such delicacies as spinach spaghetti with salami sauce, salami being one of the few meats she could drive down from New York without any refrigeration.

In this kind of work, her disability helped, she told me, since it gave her credibility with kids who were struggling with challenges of their own. Her message to them was, "Maybe you have to do it in a different way, but in one way or another you can do it." She added, "I think that was an advantage: I wasn't a regular person. I was shocked, but I learned a lot, and I hope that I opened some doors for those kids."

Later, Clipsham got involved in the antiwar movement, even taking part in Abbie Hoffman's memorable attempt to levitate the Pentagon. Eventually, though, the radical politics of the 1960s became corrupted, both without — through FBI infiltration — and within. All these years later, she remains disgusted that when Stokely Carmichael, the leader of the radical Student Nonviolent Coordinating Committee, was asked about the position of women in the movement, he replied, "Prone." Clipsham returned to making art, teaching at the Brooklyn Museum, and, increasingly, involving herself with disability issues. Among her projects was helping to oversee the design of disability-access symbols for the National Endowment for the Arts, where she was, as she puts it, "the token crip."

During this time, Clipsham had her first encounter with Little People of America. It was, she said, "a disaster." She was having trouble parking her van, and she took her case to New York City's human-rights commission. She decided to see whether LPA could offer any help. "I got the phone number of some people in LPA, some president or something," she recalled. "Called him up. The guy said, 'Are you a member of LPA?' I said, 'No,' and he said, 'Then I'm not talking to you,' and slammed the phone down." Later encounters with LPA were no better. She found the members she met to be anti-intellectual, hostile to ideas, more interested in drinking and socializing than in pushing for basic rights.

Clipsham has two broad criticisms of what she sees as LPA's view of the world. First, LPA historically has not considered dwarfism to be a disability, although that has changed in recent years, as Clipsham herself acknowledges. The second — and something she expresses with quite a bit more vehemence — is what she regards as LPA's embrace of an identity that is less than fully human. This begins with what dwarfs call themselves. Clipsham despises the word *midget,* as do most people in the dwarf community. Nor is she crazy about *dwarf* (she prefers *short statured*), although she reluctantly accepts it. What drives her over the edge, though, is *little people.*

"How do you present yourself for a job? How do you present yourself in the world?" Clipsham asked rhetorically. "If you call yourself a 'little person' — what self-respecting person calls herself a 'little woman'? I've said, 'You change your name, I'll be there.' It is very significant that you present yourself as an adult so that you can demand to be *treated* as an adult." This attitude, she believes, carries over to popular culture, where she sees depictions that infantilize dwarfs still further. She expresses a mixture of horror and contempt at people in the dwarf community who have nice things to say, for example, about Disney's *Snow White and the Seven Dwarfs.*

"They had no sex, they're . . . *happy* all the time," she told me. "And they didn't get to sleep with Snow White. The prince did. What is this? It's not mental health. And it goes back to what they call themselves, and I think that's significant. The refusal to take this issue seriously, I think, has implications for the future. It has implications for how people present themselves. And think of the damage they're doing to these children."

I'm sympathetic to Clipsham's views — she is, after all, visualizing a world that will accept my daughter as fully human, fully adult, fully competent, fully equal. But I can't accept them entirely. Ruth Ricker — who did much to move Little People of America into the mainstream of the disability-rights movement, and for whom Clipsham herself expresses considerable esteem — collects dwarf-related paraphernalia, including toys from the dreaded *Snow White.* And I've heard highly successful people with dwarfism — business people, engineers, artists — refer to themselves as *little people* without embarrassment, and without any diminution of how either they or others regard them. In a community in which debates over terminology can be outright toxic, *little people* remains the most widely accepted term.

When Becky was younger and just starting to figure out what it meant to be a dwarf, she loved *Snow White and the Seven Dwarfs.* But she was confused by the depiction of the little men, telling us that *she* certainly wasn't like any of them. *Of course not,* we assured her. *It's a cartoon. A movie. There are no such things as evil queens, either.* That was enough.

Clipsham's views are valuable for the way they expose the hypocrisy and rationalizations that often underlie the ways we think and about how that affects our behavior. But as Freud once said, sometimes a cigar is just a cigar. And sometimes a cartoon is just a cartoon.

According to the sociologist Erving Goffman, a person who carries a stigma tends to look for people who are even more stigmatized so that he can regard himself as being closer to normal than he otherwise might. "Thus do the hard of hearing stoutly see themselves as anything but deaf persons, and those with defective vision, anything but blind," Goffman writes. It's easy to see how this applies within the dwarf community. It is not unusual for LPs (insider shorthand for *little people*) to see themselves as not being disabled at all — to draw sharp distinctions between themselves and, say, the blind, the deaf, and those who use wheelchairs.

Len Sawisch, the Michigan psychologist who's also a dwarf, calls this the "thank God" technique: "Thank God you can see, thank God you can hear, thank God you're not mentally retarded." There is an intramural aspect to this as well — a kind of LP one-upmanship in which, say, a healthy achondroplastic dwarf will consider herself more fortunate than (and, by implication, superior to) a diastrophic dwarf who uses a scooter and crutches; the diastrophic, in turn, will consider himself lucky in comparison to a woman whose short stature is caused by osteogenesis imperfecta, and whose fragile bones require her to use a wheelchair.

Goffman also writes about how difficult it can be for anyone with a stigma to be treated as — or, for that matter, to behave as — anything other than a stereotype when he's in the company of "normals," a phenomenon he calls "minstrelization." (He quotes another writer, Finn Carling, who in his 1963 book, *And Yet We Are Human*, says that "the crippled" are expected to act "inferior to themselves," to "play the part of the cripple," lest the able-bodied be somehow disturbed and forced to rethink their own sense of identity. Carling continues:

> I once knew a dwarf who was a very pathetic example of this, indeed. She was very small, about four feet tall, and she was extremely well educated. In front of people, however, she was very careful not to be anything other than "the dwarf," and she played the part of the fool with the same mocking laughter and the same quick, funny movements that have been the characteristics of fools ever since the royal courts of the Middle Ages. Only when she was among friends, she could throw away her cap and bells and dare to be the woman she really was: intelligent, sad, and very lonely.

I'm not surprised that Erving Goffman is a favorite of Jacki Clipsham's, and that Len Sawisch, too, brought up his name without any prompting on my part. Ultimately what Goffman was writing about is the formation of individuality: how we create our identities, and how someone who is not regarded as the same as everyone else can create an identity that is healthy, self-regarding, unique.

The issue of identity is crucial, because it determines how LPs are seen in the world — as *dwarfs*, or as *people* with dwarfism. Unlike some parents, who are uncomfortable with the noun and who thus prefer to refer to their LP child has "having a type of dwarfism," I don't hesitate to use the label *dwarf* when describing Becky. But the reason I'm able to make a judgment like that is that I *expect* Becky to be treated as a person. And, for the most part, she has been, and is. She is a dwarf, *and* she is a person with dwarfism; to me, the two ideas are synonyms, not antonyms. Still, I recognize that my attitude toward such labeling would not be possible if it were not for some pretty incredible people — people who, unlike me, were never able to take such matters for granted.

The disability-rights movement can trace its roots to 1935, when six members of an organization called the League of the Physically Handicapped staged a sit-in in New York City to protest their exclusion from jobs in the Depression-era Works Progress Administration (WPA). The following year, thirty-five members traveled to Washington, appealing to President Franklin Roosevelt — who was, after all, disabled himself — and occupying the offices of the WPA. In 1937 they returned and, joined by the League for the Advancement of the Deaf, slept on the lawn of the WPA and the grounds of the Washington Monument. By 1938, though, the movement began to fall apart, as its more prominent activists took jobs in government and its remaining members were worn down by critics who claimed that they were communists or communist dupes.

After World War II, disability entered the American consciousness in a serious way. Medical advances meant that disabled veterans not only survived but wished to contribute to society. An important cultural moment was when Harold Russell, a sailor who had lost both of his arms, won an Oscar for his role in the 1946 movie *The Best Years of Our Lives*. President Harry Truman set up a commission to promote the hiring of disabled people, and public-service advertisements appealed directly to employers: "It's good business to hire the handicapped. How about making it *your* business, America?"

But the images of disability that predominated in the postwar era were not those of independent adults making a living. Rather, the disabled child — the poster child, an object of pity and charity — became an indispensable tool for raising funds to prevent others like her from being born. Cyndi Jones, paralyzed from polio, was a poster child for the March of Dimes when she was growing up in St. Louis. She later became the publisher and editor of *Mainstream*, a disability magazine. She once told the journalist Joseph Shapiro, author of the landmark disability-rights history *No Pity*, how special she felt when she was dressed up and photographed for the March of Dimes — a feeling that dissipated into tears when, as a first-grader, she and her classmates were handed fliers with a photograph of two healthy children labeled "This," and a photo of her on her crutches labeled "Not This." Jones told Shapiro, "The poster child says it's not okay to be disabled. It plays on fear. It says this could happen to you, your child, or your grandchild. But it says, if you just donate some money, the disabled children will go away."

Later, the poster child gave way to what is derisively known as the "supercrip" — a disabled person who performs extraordinary physical feats, such as Mark Wellman, a paraplegic mountain-climber, and Terry Fox, who lost a leg to cancer and became famous for running across Canada on an artificial limb. Wellman and Fox obviously deserve the accolades they received, but the underlying message is that the only way the disabled can receive respect instead of pity is to do things that even most able-bodied people would not attempt. Applauding Mark Wellman for pulling his paralyzed body up mountains is a lot easier, and more psychically gratifying, than making sure that city buses can accommodate wheelchairs so that non-mountain-climbing paraplegics can get to work.

By most accounts, the key moment in galvanizing the disability-rights movement — the Selma, the Stonewall, of a new consciousness — came in 1977, when a small but determined group of activists seized on an obscure federal law known as Section 504. Slipped into the Rehabilitation Act of 1973, Section 504 included a provision that prohibited federal agencies and all institutions that received federal money — such as public universities — from discriminating "solely by reason of . . . handicap."

Hardly anyone noticed that the law had been passed, and neither the president who signed it into law, Richard Nixon, nor his successor, Gerald Ford, was pressed to do anything about it. But Jimmy Carter, during his 1976 campaign, talked about disability issues, and thus raised the hopes of activists. And when he became president, those activists began pressuring Carter's secretary of Health, Education, and Welfare (HEW), Joseph Califano, to fulfill the promise of 504. The American Coalition of Citizens with Disabilities took over HEW's San Francisco office, chanted "Sign or resign!" in Califano's Washington office, and generally made themselves known in a way they had never been known before. At one point they even picketed Califano's house; Califano later recalled not daring to take his dog out for a walk for fear that his pooch would bite a disabled protester, the ultimate public-relations nightmare. Eventually, though, he agreed to enforce 504 — an enormous victory for disability rights.

One of the leaders of the 504 protest movement was Judy Heumann, whose childhood polio had left her a quadriplegic; she later became an official in the U.S. Department of Education. In an interview with Joseph Shapiro, she explained the new consciousness this way: "Disability only becomes a tragedy for me when society fails to provide the things we need to lead our lives — job opportunities or barrier-free buildings, for example. It is not a tragedy to me that I'm living in a wheelchair."

The battle over 504 touched off a string of victories that culminated in the Americans with Disabilities Act, or ADA, during the presidency of George H. W. Bush. "Let the shameful wall of exclusion finally come tumbling down," the president said at the signing ceremony, held on the South Lawn of the White House on July 26, 1990. "America welcomes into the mainstream of life all of our fellow citizens with disabilities. We embrace you for your abilities and for your disabilities, for our similarities and indeed for our differences." As Bush's remarks suggest, the ADA represented not just assistance for the disabled, but a new recognition that they are as capable of independence as the rest of society. The images of the poster child and the supercrip were replaced with those of ordinary people who wished to be treated as equal members of society. Rather than seeking charity, they demanded rights.

As has invariably been the case, dwarfs were not seen as part of this new disability consciousness. They were simply seen as being different. During World War II, for instance, little people were hired by the Ford Motor Company to work on the B-24 bomber in Willow Run, Michigan; their size made it easier for them to work inside wings and fuel cells than it was for their average-size peers. *Solidarity* magazine, published by the United Auto Workers, told their story several years ago and included photos of dwarf workers with Henry Ford, Vice President Henry Wallace, and the flying legend Eddie Rickenbacker.

"The war brought a lot of us out of show business and into factory work," said Robert Hardy, who as a youth had played the drums in a group called Rose's Midgets. "The people running the plants discovered that little people could work, just like other people. I'm glad I had that opportunity." What's significant about this is not the idea that dwarfs could work in factories, just like average-size people, but, rather, that it took an extraordinary crisis to create an opportunity. They may not have seen themselves as disabled, but society did — as socially disabled, out of the mainstream, safe to shun and exclude. In this way they shared more with women, another group that enjoyed greater job opportunities during wartime, than with other people with disabilities.

Another twist on the ambiguous relationship between dwarfism and disability can be seen in the career of Paul Steven Miller, a lawyer who is well known for his work on behalf of disability rights. Miller, a Clinton appointee to the Equal Employment Opportunity Commission (EEOC), whose term expires in mid-2004, is an achondroplastic dwarf, but his advocacy work has had little to do with dwarfism. Yet Miller learned about dwarfism as a social disability early on: despite graduating near the top of his class at Harvard Law School, he interviewed with forty-five law firms without getting a single offer.

"I was basically told by one of the lawyers at one firm that even though they didn't have a problem with my size, they thought that their clients would think they were running a circus freak show if I was a lawyer in their firm," Miller told me. I was so taken aback that I asked if the lawyer had really said that. "Yeah," Miller replied evenly. "At that time it was before the passage of the ADA, it was before it was really illegal. And people were much less subtle about it."

Eventually, Miller found work with a law firm in Los Angeles and got caught up in the disability-rights movement when he became director of litigation for the nonprofit Western Law Center for Disability Rights. His most famous client was a television news anchor named Bree Walker Lampley, who had a mild disability known as ectrodactyly, in which the bones of the fingers and toes are partially fused. A person with this condition appears to have webbed hands and feet, although in Walker Lampley's case it did not so much as prevent her from using a typewriter.

Miller became involved when a radio talk-show host and her ill-informed callers blasted Walker Lampley for becoming pregnant with a child who might also have ectrodactyly. One caller — a Claire from Oceanside — ignorantly ranted, "I would rather not be alive than have a disease like that." With Miller's help, Walker Lampley filed a complaint with the Federal Communications Commission, charging that the station had violated the terms of its license by spreading hate. The case ultimately failed, but she and Miller had made their point. And Walker Lampley gave birth to a healthy son who, like her, had ectrodactyly.

Much of Miller's practice sounds considerably more routine by today's standards, but it was groundbreaking in the 1980s — architectural access cases, school and job discrimination, suing the California state government and local officials. "It was tremendously exciting for me and the others at the center," he told me, "because we were just making it up as we went along."

Miller served on Bill Clinton's transition team in 1992 and worked as a White House liaison to the disability community until 1994, when Clinton named him to the EEOC, which enforces federal discrimination laws. On the day that I met him, at LPA's 2002 national conference in Salt Lake City, he had just finished a breakfast meeting with the chief justice of Utah's state supreme court. That evening, he would become the third recipient — and the first LP — to receive LPA's Award for Promoting Awareness of Individuals with Dwarfism. Forty-one years old, balding, with owlish glasses, Miller gets around with a cane to relieve his achondroplasia-related back problems.

I asked him about his view of the relationship between dwarfism in particular and the disability-rights movement in general — a nexus where he has spent much of his life. "I think that what is beginning to happen is that the organized LPA community is really linking arms and becoming an organizational part of the greater disability community," he replied. "I think it's part and parcel of the identity of LPA changing over the past five years or so, and of LPA having, not an identity crisis, but sort of morphing its identity into something larger than the social club that it may have been a number of years ago. I think it's fair to say that LPA as an organization is not really an active player in the broader disability movement at the national level. But I think that that's the direction we're headed in." He added: "I think it would be fair to say that I have always really connected the two experiences, both in my mind and my career."

When the late Lee Kitchens, a young engineer at Texas Instruments, showed up to work one day more than forty years ago, a co-worker approached him with some exciting news. The night before, the dwarf actor Billy Barty had been a guest on the television program *This Is Your Life*. Barty had told the host, Ralph Edwards, that he was making plans for a 1960 get-together of Little People of America, an organization he had started three years earlier. Barty had hosted that first reception, in Reno, Nevada, under banners that read MIDGETS OF AMERICA, drawing twenty-one little people from nine states. The name Little People of America was proposed by Barty at the organization's first business meeting as a compromise that would be acceptable to everyone — that is, to both "midgets and dwarfs," as the official minutes of that meeting explained.

The 1960 convention — the first since Reno — was to be held in Las Vegas, with free rooms and half-price meals. Kitchens wrote to Edwards in an attempt to reach Barty. But because he had failed to make it clear that he, too, was a dwarf, he received what he recalled as a guarded response. So Kitchens tried again — and this time he got the information he needed. Unlike many of those signing up for the convention, Kitchens was not interested in the dating scene: he was already married. But he and his wife, Mary, who was also a little person (Lee, who was four feet tall, had spondyloepiphyseal dysplasia, or SED; Mary, who died before him, had an undiagnosed type of dwarfism), thought it would be good for their adopted children, both of whom were LPs — or so they thought. Their daughter had achondroplasia, but their son grew to be five-foot-seven. Both have passed away, and Lee Kitchens would describe these tragedies with typical Texas stoicism: "My son developed leukemia when he was forty, and my daughter wound up with a bad heart. Past history."

It was with some trepidation that the Kitchens family headed off to Las Vegas. "We envisioned a fleabag hotel and a greasy spoon," Kitchens told me. "We went with the attitude that we didn't need an organization like that, but it might be great for our kids, because we had grown up without something like that." Their concern only deepened when they were told that their destination, a hotel called the Hacienda, was out on the edge of town. But when they got there, they discovered that the reason for its out-of-the-way location was that it was the newest hotel in Las Vegas; the owner was a personal friend of Barty's. There were 143 people on hand — a considerable increase from Reno. And the Kitchenses came across a piece of information that paid for the trip. Lee had been paying an extra premium for life insurance because of his physical difference; in Las Vegas, he met little people who were paying the same rate as everyone else. "I went back and told my agent, 'You've got thirty days,'" Kitchens said.

Though Billy Barty, who died in 2000 at the age of seventy-six, was the founding father of Little People of America, Lee Kitchens was perhaps its most representative member. Barty was an entertainer, one of the few good-paying professions open to dwarfs at that time; Kitchens, though not much younger than Barty (he was seventy-two when I interviewed him), led a life that was far more in line with what LPA has become: a well-educated, professional group, part of the mainstream of American life. And he'd been a leading spokesman for LPA as it made the transition from sideshow novelty to a part of the broader disability-rights movement. Sadly, and quite unexpectedly, Kitchens died in May 2003 at the age of seventy-three. I feel privileged to have had a chance to meet him.

Kitchens was a quintessential Texan, and he spoke in a deep, quiet drawl. Wearing a Western-style shirt, smoking a pipe, and sitting on an electric scooter of the sort that he and his daughter-in-law sold to other little people, Kitchens spent several hours with me, reflecting on his life. He was born into a family of modest means. When he was quite young, a philanthropist paid train fare so that his parents could take him to the Mayo Clinic to repair his cleft palate, a common complication of SED. But other than that, he had what he described as a normal upbringing, with his family heeding their doctor's advice to treat Lee like any other child. Obviously there was no LPA in those days, and Kitchens told me that he never saw another little person until he was in high school. But the state treasurer of Texas for much of the 1930s was a dwarf named Charles Lockhart. Kitchens's mother obtained a photo of Lockhart and held him up as a role model.

Lee and Mary met in college. He was an engineering student at Southern Methodist University; she was attending Texas State College for Women. They were introduced through mutual acquaintances after Lee and some of his friends had traveled to the women's school to do the repairs needed to get their radio station back on the air. "One thing led to another, we had a blind date, and that's how I met my wife," Kitchens recalled. "Two years later, after we had both graduated, we got married."

Kitchens spent virtually his entire career at Texas Instruments, spanning an era of explosive progress. He had a hand in the development of the first generation of transistors, in the early 1950s; and he helped oversee the development of TI's first calculators, in the 1970s, and first personal computers, in the 1980s. He headed up operations in the Netherlands, Italy, and the Far East. He closed out his career as a professor at Texas Tech University, and he wore a watch whose face was emblazoned with a big "TT." He also served for a time as the elected mayor of Ransom Canyon, the small city near Lubbock where he lived — a campaign made easier because of his dwarfism. "It was a snap," he said, flashing his dry sense of humor.

"Everybody in town knew who I was. I had name recognition against my opponents. And that is an advantage that little people have. It works the first time. Second time, you have to run on your record."

Throughout his adult life, Kitchens was heavily involved in Little People of America. He was the first director of District Eight, which includes Texas. He served as national president of the organization from 1964 to 1966, and helped rewrite the bylaws. And he served in a variety of elected and appointed positions, using his computer expertise to set up the organization's database of nearly twenty-five thousand people with an interest in dwarfism — LPs, average-size family members, doctors, and anyone else who had contacted the organization since 1986. At the time of his death, he was vice president of membership, and he boasted that he hadn't missed a single national conference since 1960, even though he'd sometimes had to fly overseas in order to attend.

Though Kitchens, unlike Jacki Clipsham, was quite comfortable with the term *little person*, he did not disagree with her critique of LPA as having distanced itself from the disability-rights movement early on. Indeed, as someone who had been involved almost from the organization's earliest days, Kitchens, more than anyone, watched — and helped — it grow from a network of mostly entertainers, to a social club aimed at promoting job and educational opportunities, to, finally, an organization whose members understand that they can benefit by forming a common alliance with other disability groups.

In 1978, Kitchens recalled, he represented Texas at a White House conference on disability. After that, activists started the Coalition of Texans with Disabilities — an effort that resulted in such cross-disability efforts as the blind helping the mobility-impaired with their issues, and the mobility-impaired, in turn, helping the deaf.

"That's how a lot of the civil rights for disabled people have come about, by people working together," Kitchens told me. "And it took a while for LPA and little people to chime in with that. But there were a few of us that understood that, yeah, we've got to work together. We can't do it all ourselves. Some people took the attitude of, 'No, we're not disabled.' When handicapped license plates first were available, a lot of people said, 'No, I'm not handicapped.' But you're perceived as being that way, and if you're going to wear the label, you might as well take advantage of it."

Jacki Clipsham speaks of Little People of America members as being in denial — denial about being disabled, denial about how their disability has affected their lives. The myth, she says, is that dwarfs are just like everyone else. The reality is that their difference — their disability — has affected them, changing their lives, sometimes for the better, often for the worse.

During our interview Clipsham was sitting in a wooden kitchen chair, two pillows behind her, leaning forward, with her right hand pushing on the table in front of her. The effect was of someone who was trying to appear comfortable; she surely was anything but. As she has gotten older, her achondroplasia has made her life increasingly difficult. She's had five different hip-replacement surgeries. Ten years earlier, she'd had a laminectomy, a procedure to remove pieces of the vertebrae in order to relieve pressure on the spinal cord. Not enough bone was removed, she said, but she was told that the odds were long of a second laminectomy's being successful. As a result, she's had to live with it — and has been in constant pain ever since. She can't reach her higher kitchen cabinets, which are accessible only by a ladder that she can no longer climb. In addition to her pain and mobility problems, she also has a CPAP machine in her bedroom to help with sleep apnea. To Clipsham, the notion that dwarfism is not a disability is insulting.

Yet Clipsham is, if anything, even more attuned to the idea that dwarfism is a *social* disability. She is first-rate at what she does. She has a master's degree from the Cleveland Institute of Art, and her work has been exhibited on numerous occasions in such venues as the New Jersey Center for the Visual Arts, Rutgers University, the Cleveland Museum of Art, and the New York Public Library. But Clipsham was never able to get what she really wanted — a tenured faculty position at a university — and, given her qualifications, she thinks the reason is obvious.

"The job I had at the Brooklyn Museum was an adjunct job. All I was ever able to get were adjunct jobs," she said. "I applied for tenure-track jobs; I was turned down left and right. And I knew there was discrimination. I was up against the wall." Though Clipsham remains a productive artist, her income is largely derived from a trust that her father set up for her many years ago out of the belief that she would not be able to live independently. "In some respects my father was right," she said. "It would have been very difficult for me to have supported myself. And I did try."

I asked her whether she wished she had been born without achondroplasia. It's a ticklish question. Most adult dwarfs will tell you that they did when they were younger, but that they eventually came to terms with it and now see their short stature as an asset, a part of themselves that they couldn't imagine being without. Clipsham's answer was more ambiguous.

"I don't think I would have half the awareness of people who are less fortunate than I am," she told me. "I am economically fortunate. I am socially unfortunate." She paused, then continued. "I should have been a tenured teacher at a university" — and she believes she would have been had she not been born with dwarfism. And at a time when many disability-rights activists speak of "disability pride," she takes a contrary view. "I'm not either proud or ashamed of my disability," she said. "It just is."

When Jacki Clipsham speaks of the denial that many people with dwarfism have about their disability, I wonder whether I, too, am in denial. I don't think I've ever had a moment's difficulty in accepting that Becky is breathtakingly short, that she waddles, that to people who haven't spent any time around dwarfs she is — yes — *a funny-looking kid.* But that's all cosmetic, surface stuff, the sorts of things that don't really matter. It's something else entirely when I tell myself that Becky will probably avoid any major dwarfism-related medical complications, even though one such problem nearly killed her and set back her development for two years. Or that there's no reason she can't be a better student, even though constant ear infections — despite the best efforts of Michael Cunningham, her ear-nose-and-throat doctor — have left her with a slight hearing loss and a related learning disability. Or that she can be anything she wants to be, even though I know she'll face discrimination, ostracization, and, on occasion, mockery.

Becky isn't just short — she's disabled. Recognizing that can only help her. To be in denial about the challenges she faces is to settle for less than she deserves as a full and equal member of the culture in which she finds herself.

It just is.

Chapter Seven

On Her Own Two Feet

The way I respond to a stressful situation is by removing myself from it, by intellectualizing it, by thinking about its long-term implications while refusing to look at what's right in front of me. That's how I handled — or, rather, didn't handle — my parents' terminal illnesses. In Becky's case, I decided early on that there was nothing really to be upset about because, after all, *she's going to be fine.* I had a firmer grasp on the healthy, intelligent, competent adult I imagined her becoming than I did on the sick, fragile baby who was right in front of me, and who was struggling through an unhappy infancy. Rather than living in the present, I was living in an ideal future of my own design. Fortunately for her, there were others — Barbara especially — who were focused on how she was and what she needed *right now* rather than which college she should go to and what her career options might be.

Becky's recovery from the respiratory virus that had landed her in Mass General was slow and fitful, marked by frequent setbacks. Her oxygen-saturation levels were supposed to be at 98 to 99 percent. Often — usually — they were 95, 94, 93. And it was not uncommon for them to fall to 90, 89, 88, especially when she was sleeping. We'd suction excess mucus out of her trach tube, the one aspect of her trach care with which I was intimately involved. (If I hadn't learned at least that much, I couldn't even have put her in her carriage and wheeled her around the block.) She couldn't tell us what it felt like, but given how much she hated it, it must not have been good. Since she was trying to breathe *in* at the same time that we were vacuuming her tube *out*, it had to have felt like we were taking her breath away. And we'd do this once, twice, ten times an hour, depending on how congested she was. Her nurses would flip her on her tummy and lightly tap on her back, trying to loosen the secretions in her lungs and airways and get whatever was in there up and out.

Those were dark days, and they were a lot darker for Barbara than for me. I had distractions — more distractions than I could reasonably deal with, but distractions nevertheless. Just a few weeks before Becky got sick, I started teaching a course in feature writing at Boston College. Less than a year before that I'd been promoted to managing editor of the *Phoenix*. My managers and fellow employees were wonderful during this time, but the unpalatable truth was that I was happier ensconced in my corner of the newsroom than at home or in the hospital, dealing with the needs of a sick baby, an exhausted wife, and a toddler son who was beginning to wonder where he fit in.

Barbara had few such distractions. Thanks to the home nurses that the Kaleigh Mulligan program had agreed to pay for, she was able to continue her two-days-a-week job as a photographer for the *Beverly Times*. But other than that, all of the hardships and heartaches of balancing the care of a chronically ill baby and a healthy two-year-old fell on her. I don't mean to exaggerate. The amount of nursing assistance we received was extraordinarily generous, especially during the first six months or so, and because of that Tim was able to get about as much attention as he would have if his little sister had been healthy. But psychologically, emotionally, Barbara was at Becky's bedside at all times, regardless of where her actual physical location happened to be. It was she who was Becky's extra nurse, performing most of the suctioning and all of the more advanced aspects of tracheostomy care. It was she who could tell that Becky didn't look right, didn't act right, didn't feel right. My memory is that Becky had her ups and downs during that first year with the trach; Barbara's memory, which I'm sure is more accurate than mine, is that Becky was sick practically all the time.

We celebrated Becky's first birthday in her bedroom, a large space on the first floor of our house that we had converted into a virtual hospital ward. The party took place on a stifling afternoon right before Labor Day, one of those airless late-August days when you're so sick of summer that you just want it to be over with. We cranked up the air conditioner and shut the door; heat and humidity interfered with Becky's breathing, and that was compounded by the fact that dwarf kids, for some unknown reason, tend to get hot easily. The body heat emanating from the handful of friends and family members who'd gathered in her room didn't help. Becky was hot, cranky, and tired. She couldn't quite sit on her own yet, so Barbara had propped her up in her high chair, towels stuffed strategically to keep her from keeling over. At this point, we rarely risked letting her try to breathe on her own, so the translucent blue hose that brought oxygen and moisture to her trach site was firmly in place. We put some cake in front of her, which she promptly smeared all over herself. She smiled a bit, but soon looked miserable. Then we sang "Happy Birthday." She began crying — bursts of air hissing from her trach tube to signal her distress — and the party was over.

Throughout the two years that Becky was sick and encumbered, we were encumbered, too — entangled in the arrogance and incompetence of what might be called the health-care/social-work complex. Our experience wasn't bad across the board, but it was bad enough that we were sometimes left angry, frustrated, and hurt. The home nurses were universally wonderful; the ones who were with us the longest couldn't have cared for Becky any better than if she were their own child. But the agency for which they worked often came off as an uncaring bureaucracy whose only interest was the bottom line. Every so often, the manager — a nervous, officious woman who, I'm sure, had her marching orders from her superiors — would come out for a visit, the main purpose of which was to lecture us, to remind us that we were getting a lot of services (as if we didn't know), and to warn us that eventually we would be expected to meet more of Becky's nursing needs ourselves. It sounded reasonable, I suppose, but only if you assume that the things we were using the nursing shifts for — sleeping and making a living — were unnecessary frivolities.

Once Becky's case had settled into a routine, we had an overnight nurse seven days a week, and a day nurse on Mondays and Tuesdays. Without the day nurse, Barbara would have had to quit her job. Without the night nurse, one of us would have had to stay up all night, loosening the phlegm, suctioning the trach tube, listening for the alarm whenever her oxygen sats dipped into the low 90s — as, indeed, we (well, okay, Barbara) did whenever the agency was unable to line up a night nurse, a not-uncommon occurrence, especially on weekends.

Then there was the medical-supply company. I will never forget pacing back and forth between Becky's room and the phone one day, her oxygen tank nearly empty, calling every fifteen minutes to find out where *the hell* they were with their delivery.

We were unusually lucky in one respect. Our HMO, which

managed Becky's case even though Kaleigh Mulligan was paying most of the bills, actually viewed patient advocacy as one of its missions, and it went after the supply company with admirable ferocity. I recently ran across a pathetically defensive, self-serving letter that a manager at the supply company had written to our insurer. She blamed it all on the nursing agency. No doubt she was at least partly right, given the nursing agency's shortcomings. But just rereading her letter served as a reminder of all that went wrong: a broken liquid-oxygen system; a dead battery in the portable suction machine; problems with finding an oximeter probe that would fit around Becky's unusually small toes; the company's reluctance to supply us with more than two probes a month, even though Becky was using more than that. "I have gone to the effort of reviewing the history of this patient because my name is attached to alleged statements and performance," the letter continued, all misplaced wounded feelings. "I take a great deal of pride in my work and do not want a misunderstood sequence of events to reflect substandard care."

Our insurer set us up with a different medical-supply company — and we never had another problem.

Then there was the orthopedist who walked into Becky's hospital room with a hacking cough only weeks after Becky's trach operation. We escorted her from the room. There was the occupational therapist who showed up at our home with a hacking cough, even though, presumably, she had been told about Becky's respiratory problems. We escorted *her* out the door. There was Becky's first physical therapist, who got mildly pissed off whenever Becky wanted no part of that day's session — never mind that she rarely felt well enough to take part as fully as she might have. Not only was the therapist insensitive to Becky's health, but she apparently didn't understand that kids with achondroplasia don't really *need* physical therapy; some experts go so far as to recommend against it entirely. Milestones such as sitting up, standing, and walking simply come later than they do with average-size kids, and the worst thing you can do is to push them before they're ready.

We put up with the therapist because the early-intervention agency with which we had somehow been hooked up kept sending her over and because we figured the interaction would be good for Becky, as long as she wasn't challenged beyond her physical limits. But we were made to understand — I'm quite sure of this, even though it was never expressed directly — that we were lackadaisical about our child's needs, overprotective, and did not have as firm a grasp on what should be done as they, the experts, did. One day, after Barbara and I were condescended to by the early-intervention team at the agency's headquarters, we nearly pulled Becky out. Several things were made clear: our parenting skills were inadequate; Becky's lack of progress was somehow our fault; and that, by God, we'd better shape up. If we hadn't liked Becky's speech therapist and hadn't wanted to embarrass ourselves in front of her, I'm quite sure we would have told them off right on the spot.

The bottom came later that fall and winter. On a gray weekend day in October, I was driving Tim, Becky, and two other kids whose parents we were friendly with to a roadside farm in Ipswich, maybe twenty minutes from our home, to buy pumpkins, eat apple-cider donuts, and look at the barnyard animals. Becky had even more mucus than usual, and I had to pull the car over a couple of times on the way so that I could suction her out. I guess I didn't make too much of it, or I would have turned around and headed home. But that night, she slid downhill, her oxygen-saturation numbers dropping below 90 despite the best efforts of her nurse. The next day, it was back to the PICU at Mass General, where she spent several days. She recovered, though, and she was home by the end of the week.

Then, the week before Christmas, it happened again. This time we acted more quickly and got her to Mass General before she got as sick. We have photos of her during this time, a board strapped to her arm, tubes, wires, the trach hose — and yet she's sitting up, something she'd been doing for several months by then, looking at the camera, and smiling, the upturned corners of her mouth visible beneath her pacifier. Santa Claus visited the children's floor, and we have photos of him and Becky, eyeball to eyeball. There's an unafraid curiosity in Becky's eyes, in contrast to the combination of fascination and fear with which she regarded Santa when she got a couple of years older.

Becky was released from the hospital on Friday, December 24, 1993. We were desperate to get her home before Christmas, not so much because of the holiday, but because we knew that Mass General would be all but deserted that weekend. What's the point of being in the hospital if you can't find a nurse or a doctor? Besides, Becky was definitely better. She enjoyed opening her presents on Christmas morning. With some trepidation, we even visited friends of ours with her and Timmy that afternoon. Becky kept on smiling. She obviously was happy to be out of the hospital, too.

There would be more rough times ahead, but not as rough as these. The worst was over.

Sometime in the spring of 1993, when Becky was still in the hospital, I attended my first meeting of Little People of America. Barbara was at Becky's bedside, so I strapped Tim into his car seat and drove to the Boston suburb of Newton, where a family with two boys — the older average-size, the younger achon — was hosting a meeting. There were maybe a couple of dozen people milling about. Probably ten or so were dwarfs, including Ruth Ricker, whom we had only recently met, and whom I relied on to serve as my guide into this new world.

It was, of course, a surprise to see this many little people gathered in one place. Mostly, though, I was pleased to see that nearly everyone appeared to be physically capable, gainfully employed, and reasonably happy. Talking with the parents who were hosting the event was pretty enlightening, too. Their achon son, Brian, a bright, active boy then in elementary school, had had decompression surgery on his foramen magnum when he was just a baby. It was a more serious medical problem than Becky's, yet he was running about, obviously fine. That was reassuring, but also a little scary, since I knew that Becky's respiratory woes did not exempt her from the possibility of developing other complications, including Brian's.

We made our escape just in time. There was a large bowl of Cheese Doodles that had been set out right at Tim's-eye level, and, despite my best efforts, he had scarfed down a fearsome quantity. I'm sure I don't have to tell you what happened as soon as we started driving home. At least it didn't happen on their rug.

As we became more involved in LPA, going to local meetings and reading back issues of the organization's newsletter, *LPA Today*, with which Ruth had provided us, we learned some important lessons. One of the first was a course in politically correct terminology. It's a matter of considerable controversy and debate within the dwarf community. And though I've alluded to it several times, I haven't really explained it. Now I will.

The best thing you can call our daughter is "Rebecca" or "Becky." The worst is "midget." Everything else — "little person," "LP," "dwarf," "person with dwarfism," "achon," "hey you" — falls somewhere in between. Before we started attending LPA meetings, Barbara and I would have guessed that *dwarf* and *midget* were equally offensive (or inoffensive), and that *little person*, a term with which we were vaguely aware, was probably the most acceptable. It turns out to be a whole lot more complicated than that.

Once, at an LPA parents' meeting, I heard an average-size mother say that she nearly burst into tears of rage the first time someone referred to her dwarf child as a "midget." *Why?* I wondered. Before her daughter had been born, I couldn't imagine that this mother was any more capable of parsing *dwarf* and *midget* than we had been. Within the dwarf community, the response to what is sometimes called "the M-word" is visceral; but, obviously, it is also learned. To me, it makes more sense to educate people than it does to excoriate them for a violation of political correctness that they don't even realize they're committing.

Dwarf is an ancient word dating back many centuries. In the unabridged *Oxford English Dictionary* (*OED*), the meaning of *dwarf* is straightforward and neutral: "A human being very much below the ordinary stature or size." The dictionary traces uses of the word as far back as the year 700. By contrast, *midget* was coined only in 1865, and its definition goes to the heart of why it is so deeply unpopular: "An extremely small person; *spec.* such a person publicly exhibited as a curiosity." In other words, it's impossible to think about the word *midget* without placing it within the context of the freak show, of the circus, of Midget Villages, and of Munchkins traipsing about the Land of Oz. Then, too, the root of *midget* is *midge.* And as the short-statured artist Jacki Clipsham puts it, "A midge is a small insect that can be killed with impunity."

For some reason, *midget* has another meaning as well. It refers only to a dwarf whose limbs are in the same proportion to his body as an average-size person's — generally, to people whose short stature is the result of a hormonal deficiency rather than a genetic bone anomaly, as is the case with achondroplasia and other skeletal dysplasias. Because *midget* was coined at the height of P. T. Barnum's career, and because his most famous performers, Charles Stratton and Lavinia Warren, were proportionate dwarfs, it is often assumed that it was Barnum himself who came up with the word. There is, however, no evidence for that. The word *midget* did not appear anywhere in Barnum's 1855 autobiography, *The Life of P. T. Barnum.* In fact, he referred to Stratton repeatedly as a "dwarf."

The *OED* is cryptic as to the 1865 origin of *midget,* attributing it to "*W. Cornw. Words* in *Jrnl. R. Inst. Cornw.*" Thanks a lot! But the dictionary entry also notes that, in 1869, it was used specifically to refer to a small person in Harriet Beecher Stowe's novel *Old Town Folks*: "Now you know Parson Kendall's a little midget of a man." Stowe's usage may, in fact, be the true origin of *midget*.

I put the matter to A. H. Saxon, the author of a highly regarded biography of Barnum, and, like Barnum and Stowe, a lifelong resident of Connecticut. He wrote back:

> As to Barnum, to the best of my knowledge he did *not* coin the term "midget" &, as you know, used the word *"dwarf"* when referring to the Thumbs, Nutt, &c. I have seen him use the word "midget" in a few of his letters written toward the end of his life — the 1880s — but he must have picked it up from someone else. He was a great reader, of course, & knew the Beechers.

The deep unpopularity of the M-word is a fairly recent phenomenon. Indeed, in the freak shows of the nineteenth and early twentieth centuries, *dwarf* had a more negative connotation than *midget*, according to the historian Robert Bogdan, because dwarfs were farther down the pecking order, and were assigned more degrading roles:

> The terms *midget* and *dwarf* had important social meaning in the amusement world. Small people who were well proportioned — "perfect humans in miniature" — in particular coveted the term *midget* for themselves as a way of disaffiliating from the more physically deformed *dwarf* exhibits. For midgets, who were typically cast in the high aggrandized mode, to be called a "dwarf" was like being called a "child": it was an insult. "Dwarfs" were associated with exotic freak or circus clown roles, and these roles "midgets" shunned.

As we have seen, the word had not fallen into disfavor even by 1957, when Billy Barty held the first get-together for dwarfs under the name "Midgets of America." And when it turned out that many of the people who showed up in Reno were disproportionate, Barty's solution was to change the name to Little People of America — not because *midget* was considered offensive, but because Barty wanted a name that both proportionate and disproportionate members, midgets and dwarfs, could accept. Soon, *little people* became the preferred term.

It's understandable why the newly empowered dwarf community settled on *little people*: it's safe, benign, euphemistic, coined at a time when people *liked* euphemisms. What's not entirely clear, though, is why *dwarf* eventually made a comeback, whereas *midget* slid into unacceptability. Certainly a lot of it has to do with the idea of being displayed in public. *Dwarf* is harsh, guttural, but its origins are less emotionally charged. Still, it took a younger, more politically active, in-your-face generation to popularize its use. Len Sawisch, who was involved in the creation of the Dwarf Athletic Association of America in the 1980s, says that the use of the D-word was initially quite controversial. Angela Muir Van Etten told me that the title of her 1988 autobiography, *Dwarfs Don't Live in Doll Houses*, was so unpopular among some LPA members that she thinks it hurt sales. But *dwarf* slowly grew in acceptance to the point at which, today, it's probably more popular with people under, say, fifty than *little person* is. In the 1990s some younger activists even took a stab at changing the name of LPA to reflect this new consciousness, with the American Association of People with Dwarfism being a typical suggestion. The matter was dropped because too many older members were still uncomfortable with *dwarf*. But the *little person* legacy remains something of a sore spot.

"I think that *little person*, to an intellectual, sounds very derogatory," says Matt Roloff, the current president of LPA. "It sounds more derogatory than the word *midget.* Just instinctively, people think *little person* would be a demeaning term." Adds Sawisch: "*Little people* is just euphemistic crap. If I had anything to say about it, I would get rid of the term *little people* before I'd get rid of the term *midget.* My compromise as a young man was to grab ahold of the term *dwarf.*"

Certainly one reason that *dwarf* has grown in acceptance is that it is rarely used in a truly derogatory context. By contrast, *midget* is often used as an epithet, a derisive description. I think it's significant that when the intent is to put down a little person who also happens to be disproportionate, the M-word is what gets invoked, even though it supposedly pertains only to proportionate dwarfs. Think of "midget wrestling," a term that stuck even though most of the performers were achondroplastic dwarfs. In Massachusetts in the 1980s, a judge whose budget was getting squeezed over a political hiring dispute angrily referred to the then-president of the state senate, who was unusually short, as a "corrupt midget" — a nickname that stuck thanks to the gleeful efforts of a tabloid columnist.

Now the dwarf community may be slowly coming full circle, embracing *midget* as a way of lessening its sting. Danny Black, an entertainer and talent agent who is an achondroplastic dwarf, has enraged many people in LPA circles by selling T-shirts featuring such phrases as MIDGET PORN STAR and MIDGET PETTING ZOO, the latter accompanied by a cartoon of a dwarf's being patted on the head — the sort of all-too-typical encounter with the average-size world that many LPs complain bitterly about. But despite the criticism that Black engenders, his best (indeed, practically his only) customers are dwarfs. Black says he's trying to reclaim *midget* the way more politicized parts of the gay community have reclaimed *queer* and the way some parts of the African-American community have made the N-word acceptable, at least among themselves. "Resignification," he calls it, the idea being that a minority group can change what an epithet means — or *signifies* — by embracing it for its own use.

Like Jacki Clipsham, Matt Roloff, and Len Sawisch, Black is uncomfortable with *little people*. "To me, I cringe at that," he told me. "'Little' — a term of insignificance. A term meaning 'child-like,' a term meaning 'not as great as something big.' But at the same time we're going around saying, 'Think big, think big.' Are we denying something here? What's going on? Thinking big, but we're little people. You see Fisher-Price little-people toys, little-people day care. It's childlike, it's insignificance."

At the same LPA parents meeting where I heard the mother say how hurt she felt when someone called her daughter a midget, Joan Hare — a dwarf who runs the Disability Resource Center at the College of San Mateo, near San Francisco — talked about how the language of dwarfism is evolving. Her father, she said, would get quite upset whenever he heard the M-word. Yet her twenty-three-year-old daughter, Rebecca, who's also a dwarf, often uses *midget* with her friends. Like Danny Black, Joan Hare compared *midget* to *queer* and *nigger*, and talked about how gays and blacks have reclaimed those words in part to drain them of their potency.

"Once you take a word back," she said, "it has no power to hurt."

Becky never really crawled. Most kids with achondroplasia don't. Their heads are too big and heavy, and their arms and legs are too short. The closest they come to crawling is something called "snowplowing," in which a child will prop his rear end up in the air and move forward with his legs, pushing his head across the floor as though it were a plow. Becky did some of that. But her preferred form of locomotion was to sit up and pull herself forward with her legs, scrunching her butt back and forth to facilitate the process. She invariably had a huge grin on her face when she did this, and it *was* pretty funny to watch.

A few weeks before Christmas in 1994, Becky and I went to a party held by the early-intervention program in a community center in Lynn, a down-and-out city a few miles from our home. Barbara and Timmy were gone for the weekend, visiting Barbara's family in Albany. Most of the partygoers were young, apparently single mothers, mainly Latino, many of them with *their* mothers, keeping an eye on a roaming pack of toddlers. Not only was I one of the few fathers there, but Becky was one of the few kids with any obvious sort of physical difference. The early-intervention program's clients, it seemed, were mainly struggling with poverty and discrimination rather than disability. It gave me some insight into why some of the program's staff members were so arrogant, although an explanation is not the same as an excuse. I could only imagine how they condescended to these women.

Becky had come a long way by this point. Months earlier, we'd set her up with a new physical therapist at North Shore Children's Hospital, in Salem. Not only was this therapist terrific, but Becky seemed to understand that, by going to her office rather than having her come to us, she was expected to make more of an effort.

Becky rarely needed oxygen anymore, except occasionally when she was sleeping. Usually her trach tube was covered with a disposable device made of plastic, with two paper air filters on the sides; it looked sort of like the head of a tiny hammerhead shark, with the filters where the eyes would be. Increasingly, though, she was using something called a Passy-Muir valve, which let her breathe in through the trach opening, but not out. When she'd exhale, air would leave her lungs via the usual route, up her windpipe and out through her nose and mouth. This meant that her vocal cords once again were engaged. Becky still couldn't talk, and her speech therapist had gone so far as to suggest that she learn sign language, advice we rejected out of concern that it would only delay her from talking still further. But for the first time since her surgery, her voice was back. We were thrilled.

I'd brought my video camera to the party, and I fiddled with it idly as Becky and I sat on the floor, waiting for something to happen. Soon enough, something did. Becky had been trying to stand and walk for several weeks. Now she began trying again. I turned the camera on and aimed. She would lean forward from a sitting position until her forehead was touching the floor, her legs splayed out on either side — a maneuver that would be impossible for someone lacking an achon kid's loose joints and flexibility. Then, suddenly, she would pop up, stagger uneasily, and fall back down on her rear end, laughing in delight. I encouraged her to keep trying. I sensed that this might be the day, and how many parents are lucky enough to have the videotape rolling at the very moment that their child takes her first steps? Again and again she'd pop up, only to fall. This went on for maybe ten or fifteen minutes. Then it happened. She rose, balanced herself somewhat uncertainly, and started making her way toward me, left foot, right foot, one, two, one, two, until she had closed the six-foot gap that separated us. Barbara and I watched the tape recently, and you can see her getting bigger and fuzzier as she heads toward me, finally filling the screen as she dives into my lap.

After all those months of darkness, of worry, of stress, here, finally, was the little girl we always knew she would be. Becky was tough, a fighter. In those worst moments in the hospital when she had RSV, it was her sheer refusal to give in that saved her from having to be drugged into a coma and put on a respirator. She was a feisty, determined individual, struggling with the burdens of ancient genetics and the mixed blessings of modern medicine to stand up on her own, to walk into the light, to say, "Here I am." For me, it was one of those unforgettable flashes of insight. I wanted to learn to see the world as she saw it, as though through her eyes. And I knew that if I were patient enough, and humble enough, then perhaps one day I could.

She was two years and three months old — more than twice as old as an average-size kid usually is when she takes her first steps, but right on target for a child with achondroplasia. Even with everything she'd been through, her development was on schedule.

And her childhood interrupted was soon to be transformed into childhood resumed.

Chapter Eight

Stereotypes, Stigma, and Identity

It was a chance reunion. Fifteen years earlier, Neal Gillespie and David Tilbury had shared a room at St. Joseph's Hospital, in the Baltimore suburb of Towson, Maryland. Both of them had been scheduled for surgery at the hands of Dr. Steven Kopits, an orthopedist who was such a legend within the dwarf community that the *Washington Post* once called him "The Little People's God." The nuns had asked Gillespie, then in his early thirties, to look out for Tilbury, a frightened teenager. "He was apprehensive about being put in with this old guy, and I was apprehensive about being in with this kid," Gillespie recalled. He compared their relationship to that of the Odd Couple, describing Tilbury as someone who'd throw his clothes all over the room and make fun of Gillespie for brushing his teeth regularly. But they formed a bond that they renewed instantly on this mid-August afternoon at Johns Hopkins Hospital, in Baltimore.

"My nickname for him was 'Pond Scum,'" a clearly delighted Gillespie told me, making sure that Tilbury, an aspiring lawyer, had heard him. For his part, Tilbury, upon learning that his old mentor was the mayor of his hometown of Hugoton, Kansas (population 3,700), launched into a series of jibes about what kind of city would vote for a guy like him.

But joking aside, they were both at Johns Hopkins that day on serious business. Kopits had died several months earlier following a long battle with brain cancer. They had come to see Dr. Michael Ain, an orthopedist who, at just forty-one years of age, may already have succeeded Kopits as the best-known dwarfism specialist in the country. And — very much unlike the tall, courtly Kopits — Ain is himself an achondroplastic dwarf, a four-foot-three surgeon who keeps up with his busy schedule at the speed of someone whose legs are twice as long as his and who plies his craft while standing atop one of several two-step stools he keeps stashed in Hopkins's operating rooms.

Ain is blunt, brash, and funny, a muscular man with a buzz cut and a firm handshake who was both a second baseman and a wrestler in his high-school (Phillips Andover Academy) and college (Brown University) days. Some people find him brusque and intimidating, especially former patients of Kopits, whose personal concern and solicitude were legendary. "Dr. Ain is technically very sound, but he has no bedside manner," Tilbury told me. Yet in watching Ain for a day and a half — an afternoon seeing kids at the Little People of America conference in Salt Lake City (as a member of LPA's medical-advisory board, he does free clinics at the national conference every year), and then for a twelve-hour-plus day of surgery and patient consultations at Hopkins — a more well-rounded picture emerged. Ain can be tough and in-your-face, and his humor might come off as grating for someone facing surgery. (At one point he explained to Gillespie why he doesn't like seeing patients in clinic. "I gotta talk. I gotta listen to your complaint," he quipped, all Long Island wise-ass shtick. "Hey, I don't want to do that. I want to operate. It's fun.") Yet his style also communicates something reassuring: *I'm tough, so you don't have to be. You're in good hands. You're going to be all right.*

It was the sort of assurance that Tilbury and Gillespie were in need of. A few months earlier Ain had fused several vertebrae in

Tilbury's unstable neck, a consequence of SED, his particular type of dwarfism. Tilbury had been in a halo — a sort of metal brace — for two months, and the indentations from the screws were still clearly visible on the sides of his forehead, even though he had been wearing a less restrictive type of halo for some time. His appointment with Ain was short and to the point: Tilbury wanted to get rid of the hardware; Ain wasn't so sure.

"We've been ahead of schedule every step of the way," Tilbury said, with Ain — a good six inches taller — towering over him.

"Yeah, because of you," Ain replied.

"I'm a fast healer."

"No, because you've been loosening your halo."

Ain then removed the halo. "You look great," he told Tilbury. "You look like a million bucks." Tilbury, who used to swim the length of a football field every day in the ocean near his home in the Miami area, asked if he could start swimming again. Ain told him yes, but only in a pool. Sit-ups? No, too much strain on the neck. "Go slow," Ain told him, reminding him of the negative consequences of his fusion surgery. "A lot of your mobility is going to be lost. We talked about that."

Later, Ain stopped in to examine Gillespie, who was at Hopkins for the first time. Gillespie has pseudoachondroplasia, a type of dwarfism that got its name because scientists believed it was similar to achondroplasia, the main exception being that facial features are unaffected. Now they know better: pseudoachondroplasia is actually more like SED, and people with the condition tend to have a lot of orthopedic complications, especially as they get older. Gillespie told me that Kopits had replaced both his hips and had corrected a "windswept" deformity — that is, one of his legs was bowed out and one was knock-kneed, so that they both were bent in the same direction. He had come to see Ain because of hip pain, and he suspected that he needed another hip replacement. But Ain wasn't so sure. "You actually have more movement in your hip than you do in your knee," he told Gillespie after examining him. Ain ordered more x-rays, and asked Gillespie to supply him with the last set that Kopits had taken so that he could do a comparison.

Gillespie also wanted to know if it was really necessary to come all the way back to Baltimore for a hip-replacement operation. Couldn't that be done just as easily back home? "We operate on more little people than anybody in the country," Ain replied, telling him that he performs surgery on 130 to 150 LPs a year, including hip work — and "it's completely different from average-stature." In addition, Ain told him, Johns Hopkins's anesthesiologists, nurses, and other medical staff members are experienced in working with dwarfs. "That's just as important — maybe more important," Ain said. "You only have one body. And, unfortunately, a lot of times you have only one shot at it."

For Tim's third birthday, in January 1995, we took the neighborhood kids bowling. Becky didn't bowl — she'd only been walking for a few weeks. But she delighted in staggering around and soaking in the atmosphere. She'd lurch toward the alleys, and Barbara would grab her away and put her down; then she'd head right back toward the action.

I didn't know it — how could I? — but that day marked the beginning of a new phase in my relationship with Becky. There's never been any problem figuring out what to do with Tim. We could always play catch, go bike-riding, or hike either in the nearby woods or in the White Mountains of New Hampshire. With Becky, it was always harder. She couldn't do as much, and, since she also lacked Tim's verbal agility because of her hearing and language-processing problems, it was, and is, sometimes awkward to hold a conversation with her.

But it turned out there was one thing we could share, and it was something I would not have expected: sports. Becky loves bowling and miniature golf. Every so often, on a rainy afternoon, we'll head down to the local candlepin-bowling emporium and play a string or two on one of the kids' lanes, where bumpers keep the balls from rolling into the gutter. I'm not good at it, and she has beaten me — legitimately — a couple of times. She even has a framed certificate in her bedroom that I made to commemorate one of those occasions.

I like miniature golf better than bowling, and so does she. She's so ambidextrous that I sometimes have to remind her to hold the putter left-handed, which is her stronger side. But from the time she was a toddler, she has taken it seriously, lining up her putts, concentrating, and jumping up and down excitedly when the ball drops in the cup. Once she got so excited that she fell and split her head open on the jagged edge of a bolt sticking out of a bench, requiring fourteen stitches and leaving her with a one-inch scar in the middle of her forehead. She was a little leery about returning to that particular course. But she did.

I've always felt like Tim and I occupy the same world. Becky lives in a world of her own — indeed, Barbara and I have occasionally joked about "Planet Becky" to describe her obliviousness — and sometimes a strategy must be worked out in order to find a point of entry. Even when I can't find much of anything to talk about with her, I know that we can communicate on some non-verbal level at the bowling alley or over miniature golf.

This bond has taught me something else about Becky, too. She has a strong personality; she is self-contained and stubborn, and is not easily dissuaded. I don't know how this happened — how she came to be imbued with traits that will stand her in such good stead as she makes her way through a world that won't always understand her. But I do know that I have felt the same strength of character in every successful LP adult I've met. Including Michael Ain. As a patient, Becky has seen him once. I hope she's lucky enough not to see him again in that capacity. But there's a lot more to Ain than his skill with a scalpel.

Becky met Dr. Ain in the fall of 1996, not long after she had turned five. Ain and several other specialists from Johns Hopkins were visiting a Little People of America regional conference in Lowell, Massachusetts, and Barbara and I wanted them to give Becky a once-over. For all her respiratory problems, she had never actually been seen by a dwarfism doctor. For decades Hopkins, and its Greenberg Center for Skeletal Dysplasias, has enjoyed a reputation as one of the world's leading centers for the treatment of dwarfism. Dr. Victor McKusick, a pioneer in identifying different types of dwarfism, now in his eighties, remains affiliated with Hopkins. Dr. Kopits, too, was based at Hopkins for much of his career.

Barbara took Becky to a neurologist, Dr. Orest Hurko, on a Friday afternoon, and I took her to see Ain the next morning. Ain was seeing patients in a hotel room. Becky jumped up and down on a bed, laughing, while we talked. He examined her. Her back was curved, but within normal range for a kid with achondroplasia. Her legs were bowed, but so slightly (indeed, I couldn't see it) that she would not need leg-straightening surgery — a common operation for achon kids — unless the bowing got significantly worse. I liked Ain, and liked the gruff but playful way he interacted with Becky. And I knew that if she ever ran into a serious orthopedic problem, Ain was the doctor whom I wanted in the operating room.

But Ain is more than a smart, wisecracking guy and a gifted surgeon. He is also a fascinating case study in the dwarf community's quest for identity. Billy Barty might be said to be pre-modern: an unabashed entertainer who took advantage of his size to make people laugh, but who also had the intelligence and foresight to create the framework around which a community could form. People such as Lee Kitchens, Jacki Clipsham, and Paul Miller, different though they may be in many ways, are modern: they see their dwarfism as a simple fact of life, as a disability that places them within the mainstream of the disability-rights movement. They reject the freak-show images of the past in favor of dignity and equality.

Michael Ain, by contrast, is postmodern, a man who, at various stages of his life, has ignored his own place within the dwarf community. If Barty represents dwarfism as group identity; if Kitchens, Clipsham, and Miller represent a tenuous balance between group and individual identity; then Ain represents a quest for a purely individual identity, with his dwarfism as something entirely separate from who he is as a person. I'm oversimplifying, of course; all of these categories overlap, and Ain is not the first person with dwarfism ever to succeed outside of a group context. But Ain's success says something that is particularly significant *now*, nearly fifty years after the rise of an organized dwarf community. In a world that has usually seen dwarfism — and any kind of difference — as metaphor, Ain wants you to forget the metaphor, forget the community, and consider him purely as an individual.

Ain has never attended a Little People of America conference except as a doctor. His wife is average-size; they have two young girls, one average-size, one achon. He has been frequently profiled in the media, including a segment on ABC's *20/20*, and the experience invariably leaves him with mixed feelings: he's glad to do it, but at the same time he knows it's as much because of his short stature as his surgical skills.

"I don't know if I resent it," he told me during an interview in his office after a long day of surgery and clinical appointments. "Part of it bugs me. When I was applying to medical school and residency, I caught a lot of prejudice because of my stature. And now I'm getting all this media attention *because* of my stature. I think I'm a pretty good orthopedic surgeon. And someday I'd like to get some media attention just because I did something really cool with orthopedics." He recounted the time that UPI did a story on him when he was playing second base for Brown, even though he hadn't been a starter and hadn't had a particularly good season. He knew it was because the media couldn't resist the angle of a four-foot-three baseball player. "I didn't want to do that interview, either. I don't enjoy it," he said. "I'm a fairly private person, and my private life is my private life."

When I pointed out that I was doing the same thing, interviewing him as much because of his dwarfism as his skills as a surgeon, he rolled his eyes and replied, "I might *look* stupid" — then quickly added, "I'm just teasing."

Ain seeks to be an individual in a culture that sees dwarfs as dwarfs first, people second. And for all the real progress that has been made in recent decades, the main difference is in our changing *perception* of group identity — not in a *diminution* of group identity, which would allow us to focus more clearly on the individual. Yes, Michael Ain is a dwarf. But a more important truth is that he is a person — a *person with dwarfism*, to use that phrase again. Despite some hurdles placed in his path because of his dwarfism, he is a success, respected for his skill, sought out by dwarf and non-dwarf patients alike. Yet the tendency is to see him as a Positive Role Model more than an ordinary person who likes to golf and tell bad jokes in the operating room.

There's nothing wrong with being a good role model, obviously. But to elevate Ain because of his genetic difference is as dehumanizing, in a way, as it would be to denigrate him for it.

For anyone who's part of what the sociologist Erving Goffman calls a "stigmatized group," identity as part of that group can all too easily take precedence over individual identity. Our changing attitudes toward dwarfism can be seen through artistic representations. Mini-Me and the late Hank the Angry, Drunken Dwarf aside, these representations are considerably more enlightened than they used to be. But the individual within is rarely shown, and even when he is, it is strictly within the confines of a group context.

Not long ago I rented the 1932 film *Freaks*, directed by the horror-movie pioneer Tod Browning. *Freaks* is a monumentally bad movie, and it was considered so offensive in its day that it was virtually impossible to see for many decades, excoriated in the United States and actually banned in Britain. Yet what fascinated me most was not its exploitive nature, which I had expected, but Browning's apparent good intentions. At the beginning of the film, we are told that "freaks" — that is, the disabled freak-show actors who made up much of the cast — are as human as anyone else. And in fact, the first two-thirds of the movie consists of such folks as proportionate dwarfs, an achondroplastic dwarf, mentally retarded microcephalics ("pinheads," as they were known; think of Bill Griffith's cartoon strip *Zippy the Pinhead*), and people without any limbs, all of them going about their business as normally as possible. It's voyeuristic yet progressive at the same time.

Later, though, the movie transforms itself into the nightmarish vision of disability that the earlier images seem designed to counteract. When the average-size trapeze artist and her strongman boyfriend attempt to poison the dwarf she had married for his inheritance, the "freaks" murder the boyfriend and mutilate the bride, turning her into a monster that is part-woman, part-chicken. (Like I said, it's a bad movie.) As the critic Joan Hawkins observes, the dénouement "directly contradicts the argument for tolerance that we are given at the beginning of the film. Having been initially reminded by the barker that physical difference is an 'accident of birth,' not the visible sign of some inner monstrosity, we are ultimately presented with a woman who has been turned into a freak as punishment for her immorality and greed." Browning tells us that difference is morally neutral; then he shows us that it's anything but.

One night when Becky was still a baby, we rented an Argentine film called *De eso no se habla* ("I Don't Want to Talk About It"), a 1994 movie directed by Maria Luisa Bemberg. One of the stars is an achondroplastic woman named Alejandra Podesta, who marries a mysterious stranger played by Marcello Mastraoianni. We'd heard good things about it, and for the most part we were rewarded with a well-rounded coming-of-age portrait of a young woman with dwarfism. At the end, though, she runs away from the carefully constructed life that her overbearing mother (Luisiana Brando) has built for her so that she can discover her own individuality — which she accomplishes by *joining the circus.* We see her being greeted by a circus dwarf as she embarks on her new life. The message is muddled but unmistakable: despite being well-educated, happily married, and apparently accepted by her community, she can't truly discover herself except by being with her own kind.

The modern version of this attitude was portrayed on television not too long ago, on the popular CBS show *CSI.* A murder has taken place at a Little People of America conference, and the crime-scene investigators have been called in to solve it. In the course of the next hour, we are treated to an earnest, politically correct, if not entirely accurate, seminar on the world of dwarfs and dwarfism. The dwarf actors themselves play characters who come across as capable and competent, yes, but also as prickly, defensive, bitter, even angry at their lot in life. The murderer turns out to be a dwarf who didn't want his average-size daughter to marry a dwarf man — a rather nasty bit of self-hatred that was so predictable I'm surprised it made the final cut.

I don't mean to be overly critical. The *CSI* episode stood out in many ways because of how good it was. We've certainly come a long way since *Freaks*. But I was struck by how even the most well-intentioned scriptwriters manage to fall into the trap of portraying dwarfs as associating mainly with other dwarfs (the LPA conference setting, after all, was an artistic decision, not a necessity) and as profoundly damaged by the mere fact of their dwarfism.

The one dwarf who might have been able to assert his individuality was the man who had been carrying on an affair with an average-size woman. And he was dead before the opening credits had finished rolling.

The group identity portrayed in *CSI* is clearly more progressive than that in *Freaks*, or even in *De eso no se habla*. But true individual identity is reserved for the average-size people who direct the dwarfs' lives. For the most part, the dwarfs are not actors; they are acted upon. And when they *do* act, it is in negative, even horrifying ways: to kill and mutilate, to join the circus, to plan and carry out a complicated murder in a twisted effort to negate one's own dwarfism. This is not the world in which Michael Ain resides. Or, for that matter, Martha Leo.

If Martha Leo has had a harder time than Michael Ain in persuading the world that she is somebody, that she's an individual, it's because she's had a more difficult road to travel. She's not much older than Ain; she was forty-six when we met at her apartment on a warm April morning in a dodgy, lower income neighborhood in New Haven, Connecticut. But though she hasn't attained the same type of success and recognition, her story of perseverance and of overcoming the odds is, if anything, even more impressive.

Leo has a rare type of dwarfism called SMED, an acronym for spondylometaepiphyseal dysplasia type Strudwick, which is related to SED. She stands just three-foot-two, barely coming up to my waist.

When I accepted her offer of a cup of coffee, she scampered up a massive, four-step wooden platform to get her coffeemaker. A few minutes later I watched as she kneeled on her kitchen sink and reached as high as she could to get the sugar. "One thing about being little," she quipped, "you can never say we don't get enough exercise." Fifteen cats were running around her apartment, and she made an unsuccessful attempt to persuade me to take a few home. She had recently suffered a retinal detachment in one eye, a not-uncommon complication for people with SMED. And though her vision in the other eye was fine, she was at considerable risk of a detachment in that eye, too — and, thus, of permanent blindness.

Leo lives in constant pain — so severe, she told me, that she takes methadone, a powerful narcotic normally given to heroin users trying to break their addiction. Despite all this, she is a cheerful, attractive woman with long, reddish-blond hair pulled back by a barrette. We chatted amiably for nearly two hours on her front steps, pausing only so she could acknowledge an occasional "Hi, Miss Martha!" from her predominantly African-American neighbors. Leo herself is white.

Born in Bayonne, New Jersey (she sometimes wonders if her dwarfism was caused by exposure to toxic waste), she was a sickly baby with a cleft palate who would have been left to die had her mother not insisted that her newborn child be taken out of the nursery and brought to her. But when Martha was just two, her mother — overwhelmed by her daughter's health problems and her marriage to a man whom Leo describes as an abusive alcoholic — placed her in an institution far from home, the Pine Harbor School, in rural northwestern Rhode Island. Young Martha was there for about eight years, and her memories of the place, though filled with holes, include some striking moments of clarity. Of a "wonderful nurse" named Jeannette Bruneau, who brought her Spaghettios and who later died of cancer. Of watching *Leave It to Beaver* at four-thirty every afternoon. Of kids with serious, unusual physical differences, including two who were hermaphrodites. Of playing with the only two children in the school other than her who weren't mentally retarded.

"It was so weird because you didn't know anything else," she said. "There were two kids who were pretty much normal intelligence, like myself. One kid had encephalitis as a baby, huge head. Sad. And the other one, Andrew, was just a throwaway. He was born practically on the sidewalk. He was placed there because there was no home for him. And it was the three of us. We used to dig to China — myself, Andrew, and Billy."

Leo suggested that I talk with her mother to fill in some of the missing details; but later, she told me that her mother didn't want to be interviewed. So I drove to the Providence Public Library one morning to see what I could find out about the Pine Harbor School. I learned that it was an institution housing about eighty children, who were invariably described as "retarded" or even "profoundly retarded," the presence of Martha and her friends Andrew and Billy notwithstanding. I read a story on the front page of the *Providence Journal* from 1948 that reported an eleven-year-old girl had died after having been severely scalded in a bathtub. The police ruled that the death was "[p]resumably accidental." The then-owner's lawyer told the *Journal*, "Well, go ahead and publish it if you want to. I don't intend to give the *Journal* any information." The article also noted: "The child was described in the police report as an imbecile." Martha was there from about 1957 until 1965, when the school was acquired by the Sisters of Mercy, who continued to operate it until shutting the place down in the early 1970s. Even assuming that the staff tried to do its best, it's hard to imagine a worse environment for such an intelligent, energetic child.

Fortunately, Martha had not been abandoned. Her mother, who by the mid-1960s was living in Norwalk, Connecticut, finally divorced her husband and rescued her daughter from Pine Harbor.

Martha's cleft palate was repaired when she was thirteen. And her mother undertook to mainstream her bright but barely educated daughter in a combination of private and public schools. Even though a doctor at Yale pronounced her retarded, she caught up quickly. She went to Grateful Dead concerts; she saw Bob Marley in Providence just before he died. ("At that time, he was quite sick. But he did his best.") And, against all expectations, she graduated from high school; attended Greater Hartford Community College; and then transferred to Rhode Island College, where she majored in social work and interned at a social-service agency that helped Laotian and Cambodian immigrants. "I was raised in Rhode Island, and I wanted to go back and show them I wasn't retarded," she told me. "And I did quite well."

She got her master's degree from Southern Connecticut University, walking every morning through the neighborhood that she lives in today. And she worked as a state vocational rehabilitation counselor for fourteen years, retiring in November 2001 because of a combination of mounting health problems and budget cuts that were making her job increasingly hectic and impersonal.

"I just had some serious job-performance problems," she said. "And I admit it. The last two or three years I was not doing well, and I knew it. I used to come home and cry and scream. One time I got so — I think it was one of my worst times — even my eye surgery doesn't compare to the pain I experienced that one particular day and night about the job. I came home and I knew something terrible was happening, and I couldn't figure it out, except I was not doing my job. I just couldn't function. And I cried and screamed and drank a little too much that night, to the point where my neighbors called the cops. I was out here crying away, bawling, bawling at the top of my lungs, like, losing it. Literally having a breakdown. I got juiced up pretty good, too — a little too much vodka."

There's a tendency to infantilize little people, to treat them as something other than adults with the same dreams and fantasies and desires and vices and problems as everybody else. Martha Leo, no less than Michael Ain, wants to be understood: three-foot-two or not, she is an individual, she is somebody, a somebody who's gone to Grateful Dead concerts with "long, blond hair down to my fanny," who drinks, who takes methadone, who hasn't always been a model employee. And who has sex. And who gets mildly irritated if you don't ask her about it.

"What about my love life? Little people have love lives," she said, admonishing me for my failure to ask. She plunged right in. "I don't really have any one single person now. But I was going with a guy named Dave, who is, shall we say, an urban person from the *ghet*to. He was a very strong person in my life for about four years. We lived together for about a year, and then I couldn't take it anymore. I met him at the time he was *alcoholic*, big-time, falling-down-steps kind of stuff. Threw him out the door with his bag and all, and said, 'Go get yourself together.' I'll never forget it. December 19th. *Cooold*, ice, slush, the worst day you'd ever want to put someone out. I can be very tough when I have to be. Oh, a bitch."

I asked if Dave was a dwarf. "No," she replied. "He was average-size. Unlike many of my past dates, he was about five-nine, kind of short — not real short. No, he's a normal, healthy black man. I'm attracted to black men. I don't know why, but I am. Most men I've gone with are six foot. I've always been attracted to tall men, big guys, you know? And I think it has to do with the security factor and all that, too. I don't have any stable boyfriends, shall we say. I have, like, friends who I'm comfortable with."

She batted her eyes at me and laughed. She knew exactly what she was doing. She had planted in my mind the picture of this tiny, fragile-looking white woman making passionate love with a succession of six-foot-tall black men, and she was now thoroughly enjoying my discomfited reaction.

I tried to steer the interview in another direction, asking her if she'd ever wished she wasn't a dwarf, and she told me about the time she and her mother had ripped up a Sears catalogue and its images of tall, well-proportioned women. But it was no use. All I was thinking of was her and her boyfriend in her bedroom — the one she'd showed me when I first arrived. And of her screaming at him that she'd had enough of his goddamn drinking, and that he'd damn well better get out of her house *now*.

The woman sitting next to me was a dwarf, yes. But she was an individual. She was Martha Leo. And she'd made sure that I wasn't going to forget it.

On the day before the Fourth of July in 2002, I hung out with Michael Ain in a three-room hotel suite in Salt Lake City. Several doctors were leaving for the long holiday weekend, but Ain and Kathleen "Dee" Miller — the clinical coordinator of Hopkins's Greenberg Center and, like Ain, an achondroplastic dwarf — had agreed to see a few more patients that afternoon.

We ate takeout Mexican food while waiting for the first patients to show up. Ain joked about the time that the late Jacqueline Onassis had run into him at Andover and nearly knocked him over because she had failed to look down. Later his wrestling buddy's roommate, who just happened to be John Kennedy, attempted to introduce Ain to his mother. "I said, 'I think we've met before,'" Ain told me, "and she said, 'Yeah, I think we have.' He looked at me like I had three heads. How could I have met his mother before? So it was our little secret."

I was about to see Ain at his best: interacting with children, putting them and their parents at ease while keeping them as healthy as possible. The first few cases were routine. A fourteen-year-old girl who'd been experiencing numbness when walking with a heavy backpack. (Ain told her to get a backpack with wheels.) A sixteen-year-old violin player who'd been having shoulder spasms, despite having put on an impressive display of country-style fiddling at the LPA talent show the night before. (Ain said there wasn't much he could do unless she and her parents were willing to come to Baltimore for a more thorough examination.) A sixteen-and-a-half-year-old boy who'd had spinal-fusion surgery done by Ain two years earlier. ("It looks awesome," Ain told him, adding with a laugh: "Whoever did this was really smart.")

Then came a truly scary case — scary because it underlined exactly how tenuous the health of many dwarf kids can be. Until that spring, the only achondroplasia-related problem eleven-year-old Kate Peterson had experienced was the bowing of one leg; Steven Kopits had operated on her when she was six. Then, suddenly, she lost the ability to walk, regained it, then lost it again. She and her mother, Jennifer, flew to Baltimore from their home, just outside Omaha, Nebraska, so that Ain could crack open her spinal column to relieve the pressure and then perform a spinal fusion. She walked into the hotel bedroom three months later unassisted, looking quite healthy except for a massive head brace that was held in place via a frame strapped around her chest and back. Ain told Kate and her father, Russ, that she could switch from the brace to a soft cervical collar as soon as she got home — and maybe a month or so after that, get rid of that, too.

"She should chill for the next three months," Ain told Russ Peterson, explaining, "For a fusion to be completely solid, as solid as it's going to be, is one full year." In other words, no running, no jumping, and no swimming, which Kate loved. As for the brace, Ain told her, "How about this — a year from now, drive over it with a car." Later, in the waiting room, her father told me, "She's a real brave kid. Obviously, Mom and Dad were real concerned."

The last time I saw Kate was in the hotel elevator. She and her father hadn't waited until they got home — they'd found a cervical collar in Salt Lake, and she was wearing that instead of the head brace. With the hardware gone, it was much easier to admire her head full of long braids.

"I *so* couldn't wait," she told me, obviously pleased.

My day with Ain at Johns Hopkins was different — more formal, busier, and, on the surface, at least, more dramatic. I saw him climb his step stool to perform a spinal fusion on a middle-aged achondroplastic man, lying face down, his back split open from one end to the other, Ain doing his dauntingly delicate thing while warning the anesthesiologist that the patient was starting to rouse himself. ("He's moving. You guys understand that he's moving, right?") I saw him congratulate a young surgeon for doing a good job repairing a young girl's broken elbow — then hang back so that he could discuss with him, out of my earshot, a communications breakdown that had taken place in the OR. (At least that's what I think they were talking about.) I saw him try to talk a teenage boy and his mother out of removing a tiny growth from his hand, explaining it was so small that he wasn't even sure he could find it. "Are you a tough guy or a wussie?" Ain asked the boy, putting up his small fists in mock combat. But the boy clearly wanted the growth out, so Ain gave it a try — and managed to find it, pulling out an object called a ganglion that looked like a small, elliptical marble.

Yet it was the encounter with Kate Peterson that I kept thinking about. I could see Becky in her, and her story reminded me that Becky's good health is not something that we can take for granted, not for a moment. At the end of the day, in Ain's office, surrounded by family photos and pictures, including a portrait of Theodore Roosevelt and a poster that read IT'S NOT THE SIZE OF THE DOG IN THE FIGHT, IT'S THE SIZE OF THE FIGHT IN THE DOG, I asked him how it happened that he — a guy who had always made a point of his dwarfism being unimportant — had come to take care of people like Kate Peterson and my daughter.

"Initially, I never wanted to do it," he replied, still in his green surgical scrubs, fiddling with the cap from a bottle of Poland Spring water. "When I wake up in the morning, I don't think of myself as a little person. When I go to bed at night I don't think of myself as a little person. When I want to accomplish something, or whatever, in the course of a day I never think about it. I just go out and do what I need to do to have a great day."

One day, though, he read a newspaper article about a family from Southern California who had been worried about the prospects for their achondroplastic daughter — and about how encouraged they'd felt after meeting a doctor with achondroplasia at a party. "That person was me," Ain said. "And at that point it just clicked to me that, you know, God puts us on this earth for multiple reasons. I could be a businessman. I could be a hand surgeon. I could be an engineer. But maybe — without sounding melodramatic — I could touch people's lives if I took care of little people. At that point, I decided that's what I wanted to do. And I'm pretty happy that I decided to do that." Today Ain handles 350 to 400 surgical cases a year, and about a third of those involve dwarfs.

But Ain didn't simply jump into a closer association with the dwarf world — he was pushed, too. Until he decided he wanted to become a doctor, his dwarfism had almost never been an impediment. Then he ran up against the conservative medical establishment. He applied to some thirty medical schools, and was met with rejection after rejection until, finally, he was admitted to Albany Medical College, in New York. Then he applied to fourteen residency programs, and was rejected by every one of them. Ten or so surgical residencies; ten more rejections.

"Doctors are the most shallow, closed-minded, bigoted people that I've met in my whole life," Ain told me. "It's amazing. Not all, just like there are exceptions to every rule. But these people are atrocious. And they could not see beyond their nose. They did not want to recognize that this four-foot-three individual could do the job as well as them or better. I was so angry, I was so annoyed, I was so mad I didn't know what to do." Eventually, though, he was accepted into a fellowship in orthopedic surgery at Johns Hopkins. But the pain of rejection, of being turned down repeatedly because of his group identity (an inaccurate understanding of his group identity, at that) rather than because of his individual identity, continues to smolder. His anger — and his satisfaction over his eventual triumph — is not far from the surface.

"I remember there was this doctor I met in California, where I was doing a pediatric residency," Ain said. "He was an orthopedic surgeon. I wanted to do research in orthopedics. I wanted to try to get back in the surgical field. And he told me, 'You're nuts. You'll never be a surgeon. You should just be happy and grateful that you're a pediatrician.' Nothing wrong with being a pediatrician — that's not what *he* said, that's what *I'm* saying — but, 'You should be grateful. Lucky you've gone this far.' And then with this pompous fucking attitude he said to me, 'You should thank me for this. You'll look back at this day and thank me that I told you this.' And he goes, 'What do you think?' I go — and I really said this — I said, 'Well, if I listened to every fucking asshole who told me I couldn't accomplish something because of my stature, I'd be sitting at home with my thumb up my ass.' I mean, you don't know me well, but I'm very blunt at times. I told him that. And he looked at me. And I said, 'Fuck yourself,' and I walked out of his office. And to this day he has to see me every year at the orthopedic meeting. He's got to look at me and say, 'I fucked up.' He won't apologize. He won't ever come up to me. I've only had one person apologize to me. These guys, they would never say, 'I made a mistake.'"

I was startled — as startled, in a way, as I had been four months earlier, when Martha Leo had insisted on telling me about her six-foot-tall boyfriends and her fury that had fueled the eviction of Dave, the hapless alcoholic. There was anger in Ain's voice, even rage, a gritted-teeth, controlled, *I-showed-the-bastards-anyway* type of rage that I could understand intellectually but not viscerally. Rage I won't be able to feel myself until Becky is laughed at, dismissed, rejected, and pushed aside because she's short, because she waddles, because she's not like everybody else.

Ain has a macho swagger about him, and it would be easy to say that his anger stems from not being treated like a *man*. But I don't think that's it. What he wants — demands — is to be treated like a *human being*, a person with his own individual identity, a person who just happens to belong to a group, but who is not defined by his membership in that group.

And I know that the day may come when Becky finds herself in the same position, and either overcomes her anger, as Ain did — or is overcome by it.

Chapter Nine

The Bone Machine

No one would think that Gillian Mueller is a dwarf. Twenty-seven years old at the time that we met, at a Thai restaurant near her condo in Washington, D.C., Mueller stands just a shade under five-foot-two. She tilts forward slightly and sways back and forth as she walks, but those idiosyncrasies appear to be no more than a trivial impediment — the lingering effects of a childhood accident, perhaps, or the result of a mild congenital condition.

In fact, Mueller has achondroplasia or hypochondroplasia — she's never received a definitive diagnosis — and was probably destined for a maximum height of about four-foot-two. Her extra eleven or twelve inches of height are the result of the surgeon's art: a massive, painful, and experimental undertaking in which her upper and lower leg bones were broken, external cylindrical frames known as fixators were screwed into her bones, and her legs were stretched, about a millimeter a day, to allow new bone tissue to form in the gaps. For good measure, her upper arms were stretched, too.

Mueller was the first dwarf in the United States to undergo a full course of what's called extended limb-lengthening, or ELL, which is currently the only treatment available for short-limbed dwarfism. The surgery is generally performed only on people who have achondroplasia, hypochondroplasia, and a rare type called cartilage-hair hypoplasia; most other forms of dwarfism are considered too orthopedically complicated for such drastic treatment. The day before our meeting, Mueller had helped show me around the International Center for Limb Lengthening, at Sinai Hospital of Baltimore, where Dr. Dror Paley — who operated on Mueller, and who is the best-known limb-lengthening surgeon in the country — has been based since 2001.

I had known about Mueller for a long time. After Becky's birth, one of the first articles about dwarfism that I dug up was a *People* magazine story from early 1992 on Mueller and her surgery. Titled, inevitably, "Long on Courage," the article included a picture of her with nasty-looking metal fixators surrounding and piercing her legs. *People* described the pain she went through as "often excruciating" — and yet showed an "after" photo of her lying on her back, smiling and kicking her long, normal-looking legs over her head, forcing Barbara and me to ask ourselves, *What if?* The geneticist's admonition about the horrors of limb-lengthening was still fresh. Yet here was this happy, healthy-looking teenager who was still a dwarf but who, by all outward appearances, was *not* a dwarf. Maybe this wasn't such a bad idea after all. If Becky wanted this when she was older, who were we to say no?

Two developments brought an end to our flirtation with limb-lengthening surgery. The first was Becky's two-year medical ordeal, which served to remind us that hospitals and surgery were things to avoid, not seek out, and that a healthy child was to be treasured no matter what her height. The second was our increasing involvement in Little People of America, where we met plenty of well-adjusted dwarf kids and adults who were obviously getting along in the world just fine despite their short stature.

Yet I never really forgot about Gillian Mueller. In the mid-1990s she started speaking out on the Dwarfism List, an Internet forum that I help run, defending limb-lengthening — and Dror Paley — against their numerous critics. After I posted the LPA medical-advisory board's decidedly negative statement about limb-lengthening on the organization's Web site, LPA Online, warning of such possible complications as damage to blood vessels and nerves, paralysis, arthritis, and other debilitating consequences, I agreed to post an essay she had written in defense of the procedure. And, now, here she was.

Her mother, she told me quite frankly (and thus confirming the gist of the *People* article), had pushed her into it. "My mother explained to me the differences this could make in my life," she said. "I was thirteen, I was happy. In no way was I feeling 'I hate life, I can't go around being short.' I was perfectly happy. But my mother explained to me what I would be able to do and the difficulties that were facing me in the future — driving a car, buying clothes, reaching the top shelf in a supermarket, anything like that. And I understood the functional benefits that this would have for me, and I decided it was something I should do."

Her first round of surgery, on her lower-leg bones (the tibias and fibulas), took place in the summer of 1988, right after school had gotten out, which gave her a chance to get back on her feet by September. "There was pain," she said, "but the first couple of weeks were the worst." She gained four inches in six weeks — too much — and Paley slowed her down, which reduced the pain to a manageable level. "It was never intolerable," she said. "I was never saying, 'I shouldn't have done this, get them off me.' Those thoughts never entered my mind." She took a year off from surgery, had her upper arms done in the summer of 1990, and her femurs — that is, her thighs — in the summer of 1991. By any measure, her surgery has been a success. Even her gait, though slightly off, is smoother than that of most dwarfs.

"It makes life easier," she told me. "I didn't do this for looks. I didn't care about my appearance. I mean, I care about my appearance, being neat and all that, but I didn't do this to blend in with society or to make myself appear normal when I'm not. I don't hide from the fact that I'm a little person. I did this to function."

She even runs, an activity that is at the top of any list of don'ts for dwarfs. In the past she's run as much as two to five miles a day. She admitted that Paley had advised her against it, and that her insistence on doing it anyway had already led to an operation on her right knee. Still, I often find myself thinking about the things that I love that Becky will never do: running, hiking, backpacking in the mountains. Tim and I have been heading up to the White Mountains every summer since he was nine, and I have often wished that Becky could come, too. I'm not sure it would be a good idea for Mueller to strap a twenty-pound backpack across her dwarfism-narrowed spine and head up the trail. But she certainly *looked* like she could.

To Barbara and me, major surgery with lots of pain, long periods of incapacity, and the possibility of dangerous complications is not the answer. Yet I couldn't look at Gillian without thinking of that question we had asked ourselves ten years earlier.

What if?

Gillian Mueller's recollection of how she felt about her dwarfism when she was thirteen years old struck a chord. Becky, at ten, has just begun to think about what it means to be a dwarf — to see into the future, to understand the difficulties she'll face in everything from reaching the upper shelves at the grocery store to persuading a reluctant employer that she can do the job just as well as, if not better than, anyone else. Partly this is because Barbara and I have protected her from this knowledge. Why fill her head with foreboding before she needs to face these obstacles in her daily life? Mostly it's because the realities of dwarfism, the negative aspects, are simply not a part of her life at ten the way they will be at, say, sixteen, or twenty-five, or forty.

Ten-year-olds aren't big on abstract reasoning, and Becky is no exception. We have almost never asked her to tell us her feelings about dwarfism, figuring it would be unproductive and could lead her to worry that there was something wrong with her. Recently, though, I tried. And yes, she told me that she wished she were taller, but her reasons were specific, narrow, of the moment.

I asked her if she thought there was a reason why she was a dwarf and most other people weren't.

"Because all people are different," she replied, then added: "What were they thinking when they invented dwarfs? What a dopey idea."

Why, I asked, *was it a dopey idea?*

"I already told you ten million times," she said, a rather overwrought commentary on the fact that this was the third time I had tried to ask the same question.

Tell me again.

"Make it ten million one times. One, we don't reach things without a stool or a chair. And two, we can't go on rides that we like. That's the two reasons. I told you ten million one times."

Yet it was clear, too, that she was just beginning to develop a sense of self-consciousness. Some months earlier, when she was in the third grade, New England Cable News had done a feature story on her and her "misunderstood" condition. She'd enjoyed it, recalling that she showed the reporter how she used a ruler to flip the light switch in her room. But she had refused to let the camera crew visit her school when it was in session, instead giving a guided tour after classes had gotten out for the day.

I asked her why.

"Because everyone will say, 'Becky, who's that? Becky, who's that?'" she replied. And when I asked her what would have been wrong with that, she answered, "Well, if they shoot me writing a paragraph, everyone will do *this*." She leaned forward as if mugging for the camera before adding, "Yeah, everyone will want to be on TV. So I did it after school."

A few days after the piece aired, the school principal asked if he could show a tape of it during a weekly assembly known as "family meeting." Sure, we told him, after Becky let us know that it was fine with her. Yet, all these months later, she remembered it as a moment of intense discomfort. Why? "Because forty kids and all the teachers watched it. And it was really embarrassing. I was scared at first — you know, showing the video and all that. But it felt good," she said.

You felt good?

"Well, a little. Everyone wasn't laughing at me."

But it turned out that the most intense source of embarrassment for her was a chair — a special chair that Barbara had learned about through another LPA mother. It was made of blond wood and was adjustable, with a footrest, so that her legs wouldn't dangle and fall asleep. She'd been using it since the first grade. Recently, though, she'd stopped — something I wasn't aware of until she told me during our talk.

"I got rid of my old chair," she said, quite proud of herself. "I have a regular chair like all the others, and put a stool under my desk for my feet."

You're not using that special chair anymore?

"Yeah. Good thing I have brains."

Why did you do that?

"I thought it would be brilliant. And it *is* brilliant."

Yes it is. And so is she. It won't be too many years, though, before she understands far better than she does now that it's not just her chair that looks wrong to her peers — it's *she* who looks wrong. Becky is brimming with self-esteem, but until now that has never been challenged in any significant way. We've all seen happy, energetic kids turn into sullen teenagers. They have entered the culture of adolescence, in which each person seeks to demonstrate his individuality by being just like everyone else. We have no doubt that it will be the most difficult challenge Becky has faced — more difficult, in a way, than the medical problems she had as a baby.

Becky can't be like everybody else. She already knows that, and soon she'll feel it in ways that she — and we — can't imagine. Gillian Mueller's family chose one answer to that dilemma. Our answer — one we hope Becky will eventually embrace herself — is to see her difference as a positive, as something good and distinctive, despite the pain and prejudice that she will sometimes experience.

"Because," as she said, "all people are different."

America today is a multicultural society. This multiculturalism is a tenuous thing, always in danger of being riven by those who wish to return to 1950s conformity on the one hand and by those who attack any deviation from militant political correctness on the other. But for the most part it works. It's never been easier to be different, and to embrace a non-mainstream identity, than it is in the United States, right here, right now.

But *easier* isn't the same as *easy*. And there's a countervailing force at work, too. Just as there's never been a better time or place to embrace one's identity, there's also never been a better time or place to *change* one's identity. Identity has become fluid, malleable, whatever you want it to be. Women can have bigger breasts. Men can have longer penises. Michael Jackson has transformed himself from a black man into someone who looks a white woman, albeit one from another planet.

These examples may seem trivial, but that's only because they represent the limits of what is now possible — or was, until recently. Already the unimaginable is becoming routine. For more than a century, deaf people struggled to form a community. They largely succeeded. One Sunday morning, our church "heard" a moving presentation by a deaf woman. Her family had given her a topflight education so that she could learn to speak, which had been the goal of schools for the deaf since the late nineteenth century. But as she grew increasingly aware politically, she came to reject that mentality — and refused to talk, using sign language exclusively. Indeed, she delivered her Sunday-morning sermon in American Sign Language, with her hearing fiancé — now her husband — interpreting.

Today, though, deaf culture is threatened by cochlear implants, surgery that can allow some deaf people to hear. The most famous recipient is the radio talk-show host Rush Limbaugh, who had gone deaf in a matter of months because of a rare auto-immune-system disorder. It is far more common, though, to perform cochlear-implant surgery on young children. This has led some deaf-community activists to protest that their culture is being eliminated — even to go so far as to label it "genocide." I disagree. If we had a child who could be helped by a cochlear implant, I have no doubt that Barbara and I would choose it. And the parallels between cochlear implants and limb-lengthening are pretty obvious. I can make a defensible argument that cochlear-implant surgery is less risky and painful, and has a more positive effect on a person's quality of life, than limb-lengthening. But that's strictly a mechanistic argument: make limb-lengthening less risky and less painful, and my reasoning melts away.

What was once stigma is now identity. The disabled are perhaps the last group to embrace its difference as a source of empowerment, even pride, following in the footsteps of African-Americans, women (the majority, after all), and lesbians and gay men. And dwarfs are among the last groups of people with disabilities to accept the idea of disability.

Certainly there is something illogical in taking pride in one's deafness or paralysis or dwarfism. After all, it just *is*, and on one level it makes no sense to take pride in something over which one has no control. On another level, though, it makes eminent good sense to take pride in one's ability to function in a world made for people without disabilities, just as it makes sense for African-Americans to take pride in their ability to succeed in a society designed for the psychic comfort of those whose ancestors were European.

But advances in genetic science have led, and will continue to lead, to a redefinition of what it means to be disabled. Those advances will create many more options in choosing identity and will thus call into question its very meaning. Already, genetic screening is used to weed out fetuses with Down syndrome and many other kinds of genetic conditions. In the future, doctors may routinely edit and enhance embryonic genomes, resulting in a healthier, happier, less diverse, less interesting human race.

Oh, and did I say taller, too?

After all, among the most enduring forms of discrimination is that of the tall against the short. Paying deference to those who loom above us is among our most primal behaviors, caught up, possibly, in such instinctual, precivilized matters as which male gets to breed with the most desirable female, who leads the hunt, who is dominant, who is subservient. The journalist Ralph Keyes once recounted a conversation he had with the late Harvard paleontologist Stephen Jay Gould, who, at five-foot-eight, was right around average. Gould noted that if he were just two inches taller he would actually be considered to be on the "tallish" side. "As he said this," Keyes writes, "Gould spread his thumb and forefinger slightly apart. 'It's *that* much. It's *nothing*. It's eye level that matters — whether you're looking up or looking down. So I wonder if the angle of the sight line may not function as a cue to inferred rank.'"

Study after study has shown that taller people earn more money, that their life-insurance policies are worth more, that tall politicians are able to use their height to intimidate their shorter colleagues. (Contrary to popular belief, except in presidential politics, there is little evidence that tall candidates win more elections than short ones.) Studies have even shown that people are more likely to invade the personal space surrounding a short person than a tall person. Short men wear lifts in their shoes; short women, high heels. Influential public figures go to great lengths not to appear short. Keyes notes, for example, that Jimmy Carter, who is perhaps just slightly below average, is a master at appearing taller than he really is: he moves slowly, talks softly, and slouches a bit, all attributes of someone several inches taller than he.

What is true of the merely short appears to be true for people with dwarfism as well. A recent study by a group of scientists at the National Institutes of Health and the Johns Hopkins University Biostatistics Center found that there are considerable psychic detriments to being an achondroplastic dwarf. The team interviewed 189 people with achondroplasia and 136 close relatives of people with achondroplasia. It found that people with achondroplasia have significantly lower self-esteem than average-size family members, as well as lower income, less education, and a lower rate of marriage.

The authors note that achondroplastic dwarfs whose income was higher, who were more educated, and who attended religious services regularly had more self-esteem and a better quality of life — yet this was the flip side of the finding that the dwarfs who were surveyed were less likely to have a high income and a good education in the first place. The authors observe that achondroplastic women had better self-esteem than men, an indication of the importance that the culture places on male height. They also warned that they had no way of knowing how much of the low self-esteem that they observed was due to being four feet tall, and how much was a result of other aspects of achondroplasia, mainly chronic pain and a disproportionate appearance.

But if, as Stephen Jay Gould noted, being five-foot-eight can have the effect of making that person subservient to someone who is five-foot-ten, then that would suggest that being three-foot-ten, or four-foot-two, can make someone not just subservient, but invisible, unless she can somehow show that she's worthy in the eyes of the average-size world. For dwarfs, then, basic human dignity is not something that is automatically conferred; rather, it must be earned.

It's no wonder that some dwarfs will do just about anything to be taller — to negate their identities, to become someone new. To start over. It is an enduring part of the American mythology that each of us can be anyone we choose to be. For some dwarfs, that choice starts with a long, surgical nail being hammered into their legs, up against the bone, *tap-tap-tap,* until it breaks cleanly in two.

Erica Gunnels was sitting up in her bed at Sinai Hospital when Dr. Dror Paley stopped by to check on her. A fourteen-year-old girl with achondroplasia from Mountain Grove, Missouri, Erica had huge metal fixators around each leg, with ugly-looking metal spikes running right through the surface of her skin down to the bone beneath. She was also facing additional surgery: one of the nerves in her legs had become compressed as a side effect of the limb-lengthening process, and Paley needed to get in there to relieve the pressure. It's a common complication of limb-lengthening, Paley explained, comparing it to surgery for carpal-tunnel syndrome.

Paley doesn't deny that limb-lengthening is serious and complicated and that unanticipated problems can crop up. But he stresses that cases such as Erica's are why the surgery should only be done by experienced practitioners. He said that Dr. Gavril Abramovich Ilizarov, a Russian orthopedist who virtually invented limb-lengthening in the 1950s and 1960s, and for whom the most commonly used fixator is named, once told him that as many as 10 percent of his patients suffered permanent nerve damage from the type of compression that Erica had. By performing decompression surgery as soon as symptoms appear, Paley told me, he's been able to prevent any of his patients from incurring such damage.

I asked Erica and her mother, Gina Gunnels, why they had

sought out surgery rather than simply accepting her dwarfism as a fact of life. Erica responded with a bracing dose of sarcasm. "It would be kind of nice to drive a car with pedals, and when you sit down your feet touch the ground. And to be able to reach the shelves in stores," she told me. Like, duh.

She said she eventually hoped to add seven to ten inches to her three-foot-ten-and-a-half-inch height. Her mother added: "Everybody in town loves her. She's been on the prayer list of every church in town."

Dwarfs comprise only about 5 percent of the caseload at Sinai's International Center for Limb Lengthening. Over the past fifteen years or so, Paley and his co-director and longtime surgical partner, Dr. John Herzenberg, have operated on more than five thousand patients, around two hundred of whom were dwarfs. The vast majority of their patients come in for entirely different reasons — because one leg is longer than the other, or because they have joints that need to be rebuilt, or congenital deformities that need to be corrected. Often, Paley and Herzenberg are a parent's last hope of avoiding the amputation of one of their child's congenitally malformed limbs.

But it's dwarfs who have brought Paley the most attention, from high-toned magazines such as *The New Republic* to mass-audience television shows such as ABC's *20/20*. And it's made him a controversial figure as well.

Forty-six years old at the time we met, tall, trim, and athletic-looking, Paley moved rapidly through a long day of seeing patients in his clinic and assisting with surgery in the operating room. It was late August, just a couple of weeks before the first day of school, and many families were there to wrap up a summer of treatment. Indeed, he was so busy during this traditional downtime for physicians that a reporter and photographer for the *Baltimore Sun* were on hand to document his long day. And though most of his patients were there for various types of limb deformities, several dwarfs were seeking treatment as well.

Among Paley's dwarf patients was Kevin, a twelve-year-old from Massachusetts, who'd already had four and a half inches of lengthening and leg-straightening, and who now stood four-foot-six. His father, Jim, told me that they might stop right there, explaining, "I think by going out further than that you run into more complications." ("Kevin" and "Jim" are their real first names, but they asked that I not use their last names, or identify what community they're from.) When I related that conversation to Paley later, he laughed and said, "That's what they say now. Kevin's going to be five-foot-four, I'll bet you anything. Because they won't stop halfway. They had such a positive experience."

I watched as a teenage boy with dwarfism had the fixators removed from his legs while under general anesthesia. Paley stuck a pair of surgical scissors into each hole where the huge pins had come out and cut away at the flesh underneath. The result was a bloody mess — but Paley explained that the crude-looking procedure virtually eliminated the indented scars that many of his earlier patients have. I accompanied him as he consulted with a hypochondroplastic teenage girl and her mother; she'd had leg-lengthening done elsewhere, and had suffered nerve damage as a result. I visited with a mother and her achondroplastic son as he awaited the surgery that would begin his last round of lengthening. He was four-foot-eight — six inches taller than his anticipated natural height of four-foot-two — and she was expecting him to end up at around five-foot-four. Why do it? "To make life easy," she said. "Just like anything else in life, we take some risks to make things easy."

The vague disrepute that surrounds limb-lengthening had obviously had its effect on the families whom I met. They knew they were violating our culture's supposed embrace of diversity, and they knew their decision would be unpopular with many people — even those who might, in a similar position, do exactly the same thing. Not one of the families I talked with had ever been involved in Little People of America. Erica and Gina Gunnels were the only folks I met that day who allowed me to identify them fully. And Jim, Kevin's father, started to become angry when he perceived that my line of questioning betrayed my disapproval of the surgery.

Jim was right. To me, the surgery has too many risks, is too painful, and is too incapacitating for too long a time period. At best, it takes three summers out of a child's life — summers he will never get back. But, still, there's no question that it's a lot easier to be five feet tall than four feet. There's also no question that these parents only wanted what was best for their children — and that they had sought out one of the best doctors in the country to perform the surgery. Yes, I disapprove, but I don't condemn. Who knows? Maybe they're right and I'm wrong.

Yet there's also no question that limb-lengthening raises troublesome ethical questions, none more so than the fact that it is most effective when performed on kids in their early teens, or even younger. Paley said he's learned in the past few years that he gets the best results if he does one round of limb-lengthening between the ages of six and ten, and then does subsequent rounds when the kids reach their teens. The mother I talked with who told me she wanted to "make life easy" for her son said this when I asked her about the notion of informed consent: "I just don't think they're old enough to make this kind of big decision. This is a very high-risk operation."

By the time a child reaches her late teens, the surgery simply doesn't work as well. Thus limb-lengthening is irretrievably intertwined with the perverse reality that it is best done at an age when a child is most influenced by peer pressure, is most concerned about body image, and is obsessed with looking like everyone else. A child who might willingly — eagerly — embrace limb-lengthening at, say, twelve could have a completely different opinion by the time he is eighteen, or twenty-one, or thirty. I have talked with dozens of dwarf adults over the past ten years. Without exception, every one of them has told me that adolescence was the most difficult time for them, that they wished they weren't dwarfs, that being excluded from dating and the high-school social scene was excruciating. Yet virtually every one of them say that with age came wisdom — that, as adults, they came to realize that their dwarfism gave them a perspective and outlook they would not have had otherwise, and that they no longer had any interest in being average-size.

Then, too, a dwarf who has undergone limb-lengthening is still a dwarf. Someone with achondroplasia who marries an average-size partner still has a fifty percent chance of giving birth to a child with achondroplasia. Their spinal openings are still too small — although Paley says that, because his method of limb-lengthening also straightens the back, there is less pinching and, theoretically at least, a somewhat reduced risk of spinal-cord compression. Their hands are still tiny, their heads are still big, their faces still shine with achondroplastic features. (Gillian Mueller, who has few dwarf features, is a rare exception to this truth.) And they'll be short — not four feet tall, of course, but in many cases six or more inches shorter than average-size people. Rather than curing dwarfism, limb-lengthening can sentence those who've had it to a kind of neither-fish-nor-fowl limbo.

Dr. Michael Ain, the Johns Hopkins orthopedic surgeon who's also an achondroplastic dwarf, actually considered limb-lengthening when he was a kid. Yet he is unstinting in his criticism of the procedure and especially of the notion that parents should make such an important decision for their children. During my day with him in Baltimore, he told me he had just seen a fifteen-year-old boy who was considering the surgery. "He really had a good grasp on it, and he was old enough to make it," Ain said. "His parents weren't making it for him. I think that's a terrible thing. That's what I fight. I don't want some parent who's guilty or who has some kind of different agenda or hang-up make the decision for the child. That's a horrible thing.

He or she should understand all the risks and complications of it, from significant arthritis possibly, stiffness, nerve problems, paralysis, death — all these things. I'm not being melodramatic."

Ain added: "The complication rate is incredibly high. They've gotten better, but it's still amazingly high. John Herzenberg and Dror Paley are two of the best people. If my daughter needed limb-lengthening, I would without a doubt go to them, because I think they're fantastic in doing it. But I'm not rushing out to bang on their door and make an appointment, either."

Michael Ain's invocation of the D-word — as in "death" — drives Dror Paley up a wall. Ain didn't just use it with me; he used it when *20/20* interviewed him, when CBS interviewed him, and who knows on how many other occasions as well. "I got very upset with Michael when he was interviewed on television and they had him saying, 'You could die from this,'" Paley told me. "Yeah, so big deal, Michael, you could die from this. Tell me one operation you do where you couldn't die from it. Have any of my patients died from it? No. So why are you getting on TV and doing this sensationalism?"

Paley's right, of course, but he's wrong, too. It depends on your perspective. Death in the course of a twelve-hour spinal decompression might be a risk worth taking if the alternative is to spend the rest of your life in pain, in a wheelchair, incontinent, impotent, depressed. But is it worth it to be eight, ten, twelve inches taller? To undergo what is regarded by many people as cosmetic surgery? Paley's response: "Yeah, it's great, it's wonderful to accept yourself as a dwarf, but you know what? It's great to be a Michael Ain, but not everybody's a Michael Ain. It's a lot easier for a lot of them who aren't going to be Michael Ains to be taller. It solves a lot of problems."

During my day at Sinai, I had a chance to interview Paley's partner, John Herzenberg, as well. And he made what I thought was an important point: that a dwarf gains considerable benefit from limb-lengthening simply because his upper arms are made longer. "What is the most important thing you can think of other than being able to wipe yourself?" he asked. I don't disagree. Becky has a terrible time trying to clean up after going to the bathroom. Recently we bought her a "magic wand" — a reacher for personal hygiene that Danny Black sells — but she's having a tough time figuring out how to use it. On a less intimate note, Becky started playing the clarinet in the fourth grade — and nearly had to give it up because she couldn't reach the keys at the bottom of the instrument. Fortunately a sympathetic teacher located an E-flat soprano clarinet, which is smaller and easier for her to handle. But it was just another indication of the little ways in which life can be more difficult for a kid with dwarfism. And her problems will only get worse as she grows older and changes from a double-jointed ten-year-old to a prematurely stiff adult.

Dr. Michael Goldberg, an orthopedist at New England Medical Center, in Boston, who sees a number of dwarf patients (including Becky), has told me that he thinks it might actually make sense for dwarfs to undergo limb-lengthening on their arms, although he remains opposed to leg-lengthening on the grounds that it is too painful and dangerous, with too limited a payoff. Goldberg said that surgeons at his institution are adding maybe an inch to the upper arms of achondroplastic kids and fixing their elbows so they can straighten their arms fully. But when I asked Dr. Herzenberg whether anyone had ever come to him seeking just arm-lengthening, his reaction appeared to be one of genuine puzzlement, like the thought had never occurred to him. Obviously by the time people find their way to Paley's and Herzenberg's door, they're not interested in any half-measures. They want to be tall. Or, to be more accurate, taller.

Paley and I finally had a chance to sit down around ten o'clock at night, at a Middle Eastern restaurant in a strip mall near his home in the Baltimore suburbs. He was candid, persuasive, eloquent. An immigrant from Israel by way of Canada, he bantered with the waiter over how *hummus* is pronounced in Hebrew and Arabic. And he impressed upon me that he is absolutely sure that he is doing the right thing.

Paley studied limb-lengthening in Italy and Russia in 1986, beginning his work at the University of Maryland the following year. Herzenberg became his surgical partner in 1991, and they ran the Maryland Center for Limb Lengthening at the university until 2001, when Sinai made them the proverbial offer they couldn't refuse. They may well be the most experienced limb-lengthening surgeons in the country, and Paley said they got that way by taking all comers, not just dwarfs. He said dwarfs shouldn't even consider going to limb-lengthening surgeons whose only area of expertise is dwarfism, since they lack the wide range of experiences necessary to solve problems as they come up.

The politics of limb-lengthening within Little People of America is fraught with emotion. But it is safe to say that Paley is unpopular in LPA circles — not just because he does limb-lengthening, but because he's perceived as arrogant, a showman, a salesman. Some years ago the organization decided to recommend that those seeking the surgery have it done at Cedar-Sinai Medical Center, in Los Angeles, which was following an experimental protocol and which mandated psychological counseling for all of its prospective limb-lengthening patients. Paley expressed disdain, telling me that his method is better than the one used at Cedar-Sinai, and that he'd long ago stopped offering counseling for dwarfs. "I decided that doing psychological evaluations of teenagers had no value whatsoever," he said, laughing slightly.

But he grew more serious when he talked about what he sees as LPA's unwillingness to let him meet with members and discuss his work. Paley had actually been invited to make a presentation to the medical-advisory board at the 2002 LPA conference in Salt Lake. It never happened: the invitation was rescinded by the LPA executive committee. LPA's president, Matt Roloff, told me that the committee disinvited Paley because his presentation was scheduled to be open to the general membership, not just the medical professionals. "The official reason why he was disinvited was that they feel he is overly zealous in the marketing of ELL," Roloff said. "They were scared to death that Dr. Paley would be off in a corner recruiting people." Roloff added that he would like to see LPA become more open to the whole subject of limb-lengthening — but that he and other officers would rather hear from someone they consider to be more low-key than Paley — such as, ironically, Herzenberg.

Paley, though, labeled the withdrawal of the invitation as "narrow-minded," and disagreed with those who criticize him as a self-promoter. He doesn't seek out the media, he said; rather, they come to him. If nothing else, he added, LPA should be willing to help members find limb-lengthening surgeons with a good track record. "There were at least ten patients in clinic today who had been screwed up by other doctors," he said. "They just don't know what they're doing."

We discussed one case — briefly celebrated by the media in the 1980s — involving a young patient who had been turned away by Paley because he was simply too short and who later ran into trouble with another surgeon. "They end up getting half-assed treatments, bad treatments. That gives what I do a bad name. I don't have a single patient like that," Paley said. (I later learned that the boy, now a young adult, was involved in a $1.85 million legal case against his surgeon. I wrote to him, seeking an interview, and received a call from someone identifying himself as his brother, who told me that he was not allowed to discuss the case. The law firm that represented him did not respond to my inquiry, either.)

Yet Paley's track record is not perfect, as he himself willingly revealed. In just the past few years, he and Herzenberg have learned that dwarfs with a certain type of spinal deformity are vulnerable to spinal-cord injury when undergoing some of the procedures involved in limb-lengthening. The most extreme case involved a young woman who eventually was sent to Dr. Ain for decompression surgery and who now is partially paralyzed and walks with a cane. "To me, she's a terrible result," Paley said. "I actually don't know how she rates herself. But to me, she would have been better off if she had never had the lengthening."

So why do it? Why put dwarfs through major surgery when there's a strong case to be made that there's nothing wrong with them in the first place? Why should insurance companies lay out as much as $230,000 to pay for a full course of treatment?

"Our society is designed for easier accessibility around the height of about five feet tall, maybe even taller than that. If you're five feet tall, the height of the chair, the distance to the gas pedal in a car, the coat hanger right there — I mean, that coat hanger right there is almost inaccessible to most dwarfs," Paley replied, pointing to one behind my chair. "But who designed it to be that way? If we were all three feet tall, it wouldn't be that high, would it? The position of that handle on the door is not designed for a dwarf. It will hit him in the forehead. So he has to reach up here to hold that handle. The door knob, the light switches — it's a fact of life.

"Okay, fine. You can live as a short-statured person, but you are more challenged. And if you could safely make someone fit into the more normal height range, their life would be easier. And I think if somebody has the resources to do that — insurance, or personal funds, because it's not emergency surgery — and is willing to go through the pain and suffering and inconvenience and everything else to go through it, and you've got a caretaker who can provide it in a reasonable fashion where the risks are acceptable, then it's a reasonable thing to do. And that's my philosophy on it."

As is so often the case in such conversations, Paley was talking about dwarfism as a *socially constructed* disability, an inability to fit into the human-built environment. But is limb-lengthening the answer to that dilemma? And are those who undergo it really happier? Michael Goldberg told me that he opposes limb-lengthening not because it is unnecessary in all cases, but because, in his view, it is unnecessary in this culture. Several years ago, for instance, he helped conduct a study of how achondroplastic adults view their own physical and mental health. He found that their self-perception of physical health began to decline in comparison to that of the average-size majority once they reached their forties — the result, he suspects, of age-related orthopedic problems. Yet he found no difference in *mental* health between achondroplastic and average-size adults.

In contrast to the situation that prevails in the United States, Goldberg recalled meeting a teenager from Verona, Italy, who'd undergone limb-lengthening at the hands of Italian doctors. It had not gone terribly well; she'd suffered some sciatic-nerve damage, needed a leg brace, and had had to give up sports. Yet without the surgery, she would not have been allowed to drive a car or to attend a regular school for "normal" kids. For her, at least, Goldberg considered the operation a success, adding: "She was happy as can be."

In other words, our culture is better at accommodating disability than some others are. Doesn't it make more sense to keep changing the culture and making it even better?

After I turned my tape recorder off, as we were walking outside to our cars, Paley said something else. I wasn't taking notes, but it went pretty much like this: *Now that you've seen limb-lengthening up close, now that you know it can work and improve people's lives, don't you have an obligation to tell your daughter about it? Shouldn't she at least know that such a procedure exists? Maybe some day she'll want it for herself.*

I made a small joke about his trying to lay some guilt on me, but I did think about it. It struck me as contradictory coming from someone who, just twelve hours earlier, had told me that psychological evaluations of dwarf teenagers were worthless, that of course it's the parents who must take the lead in making the decision. Not that Paley would advocate limb-lengthening against a child's will — after all, given the pain and commitment and months of physical therapy involved, the results would be disastrous unless the patient were thoroughly on board. But if a parent can push a child into having limb-lengthening surgery, why can't he do the opposite as well: simply keep knowledge of the procedure to himself, to withhold that option?

Still, Paley had a point. Much as Barbara and I oppose limb-lengthening for Becky, if she somehow learned about it and insisted on having it done, we're not sure what we'd do. If we couldn't talk her out of it, and if her overall health made her a good candidate, I doubt that we'd refuse.

Just before writing this, I showed Becky a videotape of a twelve-and-a-half-minute feature story that CBS News had broadcast on a recent Sunday morning. It included Paley and Ain making the case for and against limb-lengthening (yes, Ain used the D-word again); the dwarf actor Danny Woodburn, who was adamantly opposed to the surgery; and several of Paley's young patients, who were shown both walking around and lying in the operating room, getting huge steel screws inserted into their legs.

I didn't say much. I told Becky that I had met both Dr. Paley and Dr. Ain, and that Ain had once examined her in a hotel room at an LPA meeting. Her response: *That looks like pain. Getting tubes put in my ears and getting shots is bad enough.* I assured her that she was fine just the way she was, that we would never push her to have such surgery, and that, in fact, we hoped she wouldn't want it.

And we *do* hope she won't want it, notwithstanding the possibility that we might talk with her about getting her arms lengthened when she's a little older. But the truth is that I have no idea of what seed I might have planted in Becky's mind by showing her that videotape.

Within days, she was telling me that she wanted to show it to her class. (Her teacher talked her out of it.)

So far, being a dwarf hasn't been much of an impediment for Becky. She's too young to drive, she's too young to date, and if she really, really needs to reach something, she can just ask Mom or Dad to grab it for her. In a few years, though, she no doubt will have developed a full-blown critique of dwarfism, and it's not likely to be a favorable one.

We wouldn't have chosen dwarfism for her. If there was a magic pill that would "cure" her of achondroplasia, we'd give it to her. But there isn't a magic pill. Limb-lengthening is an imperfect solution to a problem that is more the culture's than hers.

Besides, there is value to Becky's dwarfism — as there is to diversity, to individuality, to identity. Breaking her bones and stretching them out would call that identity into question. She would be a tall dwarf, genetically programmed to have children who are dwarfs. She would still be destined to have the same back and joint and respiratory problems that she would have had if she had only grown to be four feet tall. But now those problems would be complicated by the uncertain long-term health of surgically lengthened bones. She would be stuck between two worlds, no longer quite accepted by the dwarf community but not really part of the average-size majority, either.

As F. Scott Fitzgerald once wrote, "The test of a first-rate intelligence is the ability to hold two opposed ideas in the mind at the same time, and still retain the ability to function." Here are the two contradictory thoughts that I struggle with: Becky's genome is imperfect, and thus her life will be imperfect in ways different from — but not worse than — those of her average-size peers. And Becky is perfect just the way she is.

It's a message that she not only needs to hear, but understand and absorb as well.

CHAPTER TEN

THE STORM BEFORE THE CALM

In 1995, as winter struggled to turn into spring, we found ourselves in a kind of suspended animation. Becky was doing well, Tim continued to grow and thrive, and we were thoroughly acclimated to our home's being open to nurses and medical-supply workers at all hours of the day and night. The *Beverly Times* was switching over to a computerized photo-editing system, which meant that Barbara was putting in sixteen-hour days for a while. It was not unusual for her to arrive home after eleven o'clock at night on Mondays and Tuesdays — the two days that she worked — to find Becky's night nurse, Renée Maloney, and me laughing uproariously at *Beavis and Butt-head.*

But though it might have looked like a comfortable routine, it only masked the stress under which we were living. Every parent of a young child knows that nothing stays the same for long. That's doubly true when you're tending to the needs of a sick child.

By this point Becky was getting seventy-two hours of home nursing care each week: seven overnight shifts, plus Barbara's two work days. That was a slight reduction from the eighty-four hours we had received during the first few months after Becky's discharge from

Mass General, but it was still substantial. And we knew it would soon end. The nursing agency was already showing little ability — or inclination — to fill all of the overnight weekend shifts. And the nursing supervisor stopped by for a visit one evening to inform us that we could expect a significant cutback in our weekly schedule, since the state couldn't be expected to pay for such extravagance indefinitely. I wondered if anyone had ever talked that way to the CEOs of Fidelity Investments and Raytheon, who were receiving roughly $100 million in tax breaks from Massachusetts politicians at roughly the same time that we were being lectured to about how selfish it was to expect to sleep on a Sunday night.

Dr. Cunningham and Dr. Shannon had told us from the beginning that Becky would need her trach for about two years. She hit the second-anniversary mark in February. Barbara was already making plans to enroll Becky in preschool that fall, giving her a long overdue chance to be with other children in a normal, worry-free environment. Cunningham wanted to try to remove the trach later in the spring. If all went according to plan, Becky could begin a new life as a regular little girl. But if the trach had to stay, Cunningham had already informed us that he wouldn't try again for another year. Becky's progress would be dealt a huge setback. Fewer nursing hours meant that we — mainly Barbara — would have to choose between sleep and work. And we would remain dependent on a bureaucracy that was becoming increasingly unresponsive.

It was, in many respects, the most nerve-wracking time we'd had since those two months in Mass General. We felt like everything was hanging in the balance when Becky entered Mass Eye and Ear the first week of May to have her trach removed. Within hours, that pressure would be ratcheted up to the boiling point.

Becky was put under general anesthesia so that Dr. Cunningham could remove her trach tube, give her trachea a close look, and slice off any scar tissue and overgrowth that had built up inside. She was slow in coming around from anesthesia after her surgery. Combined with what Cunningham described as a "floppy larynx," Becky was, for many hours after decannulation (the medical term for undoing a tracheostomy), unable to breathe without something plugged into her trach hole to keep her airways open. Her trachea had done its job over the previous two years, growing to the point where she could inhale enough oxygen and exhale enough carbon dioxide — but only if there were something there to keep her airway open and prevent it from collapsing in on itself.

I saw Becky a few hours after surgery. She was sitting up in bed, watching *Winnie the Pooh* videos, with some sort of a tube with tape over the end inserted into her trach opening, not letting air in, but just holding the walls of her trachea apart. Becky was tired, unresponsive, unhappy. Cunningham explained that she struggled to breathe every time he attempted to remove the tube, that she wasn't quite ready yet, and that he hoped he'd have better luck the following day. But he made it clear that if there was no change, she'd have to keep her trach.

I drove Tim home while Barbara stayed at the hospital. It was a long, slow, terrible drive. For some reason, I have a photographic memory of looking at the cement plant that sits in the middle of the interchange joining Interstate 93 and Route 1. I have no idea why. I also recall thinking that all of our hopes and dreams were on the verge of being dashed — that Becky, who I'd always thought of as a normal kid who'd had one unusual but temporary problem, was turning into a chronically ill, disabled child who would never be all right, and that her life and our lives would forever be defined by that reality.

And yet amazingly, miraculously, the next day brought a complete turnaround. It was as simple and undramatic as this: one day she couldn't; the next day she could. As the aftereffects of the anesthesia wore off and she got her strength back, the walls of her trachea became strong enough that they could support themselves on their own. Becky came home completely unencumbered: no trach tube, no oxygen, no suctioning machine, no nothing. In less than twenty-four hours we'd hit bottom and then been vaulted to the top.

It was over. She was free. And so were we.

Removing a trach tube from a healthy toddler is not the sort of procedure that requires a lengthy recovery. Becky went from being a child with significant medical problems on May 4, 1995, to being a perfectly healthy, average kid — albeit one with dwarfism — on May 5. Because the nurses had already been scheduled for the week, we let them keep coming — after all, it would take us time to get our confidence back. For a few days we kept using the oximeter at night, taping the probe to her toe. Her oxygen-saturation levels stayed in the upper 90s. Unbelievable.

Once we began to accept that this gift was real, we did what we'd dreamed of doing for two years. We bid a tearful goodbye to the nurses. We told their supervisor that her agency's services were no longer needed — a particularly satisfying moment. We called the medical-supply company to schedule the removal of its equipment. We arranged to cancel the government benefits we'd received through the Kaleigh Mulligan program. We moved Becky upstairs, to a bedroom next to Tim's and ours, and converted her home hospital ward into a new TV room. And we had a big party for her in August, with dozens of friends and family members, complete with a huge Bouncy Bounce, an inflatable house inside which she and the other kids jumped up and down to the point of nausea. Barbara's entire family was there — her parents, John and Joan Tanski; her sister, Mary Zysinski; her brothers, Jack and Steve Tanski, and Steve's wife, Darlene; and assorted nieces and nephews.

But if Becky easily made the transition from sick to normal, it turned out to be unexpectedly hard for Barbara. For the first time, Becky wasn't completely dependent on Barbara for her every need.

Intellectually, Barbara knew she was finally free, or as free as the mother of two young children can be. Emotionally, she couldn't let go. At Dr. Cunningham's suggestion, we had asked the medical-supply company to let us keep the oximeter for one year. Every time Becky got a sniffle, Barbara hooked it up, watching the numbers and making sure everything was okay. It bothered her that if Becky's oxygen sats dropped during the night, there'd be no alarm that would go off, and thus no parent or nurse to run to her side, patting her on the back, making sure she was okay. All that was over and unnecessary now — except in Barbara's mind.

"I felt like I couldn't breathe," she told me one afternoon, remembering that difficult spring and summer. I asked her if she thought she'd been depressed. She replied that she wasn't sure; she had no basis of comparison, no previous knowledge, to know what depression felt like. What she did know was that she'd coped with the previous two years by keeping herself in crisis mode twenty-four hours a day. And that it took her a long time, weeks, months, to get *out* of crisis mode. Even seven years later, a stretch during which Becky's health has been completely normal with the exception of a steady stream of ear infections, Barbara has still not completely let go. She told me that if she's sitting in the TV room at ten or eleven at night and she hears a truck coming down the street, she instinctively relaxes and tells herself, *Okay, Renée's pulling into the driveway. I can go to bed now and stop worrying for a few hours.* I had no idea — a confession that I'm sure will sound familiar to every mother whose husband is not as fully engaged as he would like to think he is.

My guess is that Barbara had post-traumatic-stress disorder, and has a touch of it still. It's not disabling — no more than an occasional flashback, really — but it's still there in the back of her mind. Stoic to a fault, she's never talked about it with anyone but me, and then only when prodded. I can only imagine how much worse it must be for families with a child whose problems and needs are greater than

Becky's. I've tried hard not to compare Becky's — and our — problems with anyone else's. What we went through was what we went through. The fact that babies are born with fatal illnesses, that kids are paralyzed in diving accidents, or, for that matter, that families sell their daughters into prostitution on the streets of Calcutta doesn't change any of that. It dishonors Becky and trivializes what was genuinely a traumatic time in our lives to dismiss it by saying, well, it could have been a lot worse.

Even so, I can't help but feel a sense of awe when I think about families who are able to hold heart and soul together when faced with much greater challenges than we ever had to deal with — children who aren't going to get better, children who aren't going to live long, children who will never be able to return the love that their parents shower upon them every hour of every day. We got just a taste of what that must be like, and it was enough. More than enough.

We've all read about white couples who adopt a black child, or an Asian child, and then struggle to put him in touch with his ethnic heritage. They understand that it would be extraordinarily hard, and harmful, to raise their children in an all-white world, completely disconnected from others like them. Kids need to learn that we're all the same. But they must also learn what it means to be different — the good, the bad, the myths, the truths.

Dwarfism, as we've seen, is many things. It's a genetic difference. It's a disability. It's a culture with its own millennia-old history. It's an identity, an identity that can be altered, if not immutably changed, through years of painful, potentially dangerous surgery. And it's a minority group, similar in many ways to minorities such as African-Americans, Asians, Latinos, and Jews.

I know families who have traveled with their dwarf kids to the national conference of Little People of America every summer just so their children can be with other dwarfs. We haven't, although I attended the 2002 conference, in Salt Lake City, as research for this book. But we have tried to make it to regional conferences whenever we could, attending events in every New England state but Vermont. Becky didn't seem to care much about LPA one way or the other when she was younger. But it's grown increasingly important to her the past several years as she has become more aware of her dwarfism and of the reality that she's not like everyone else.

Even more than such occasional gatherings, though, I think it's important that any child who is different have the opportunity to get to know other people with the same difference, to see that their difference is not something they're going to grow out of, that they can take some pride in it, hold their heads high, and succeed in spite of it, or maybe even because of it.

For Becky, and us, that person has been Ruth Ricker. Ruth has made several cameos to this point. But she has meant far more to us than simply being an occasional presence in our lives. When Becky was sick, I looked to Ruth as a model, a real-life symbol of what Becky could be if she could just get better. When Becky got a little older and couldn't quite understand the whole dwarfism thing — that, no, she wouldn't remain a child forever just because she was shorter than everyone else — Ruth helped explain it to her, told her that she had a job, owned a home, and drove a car, just like Mom and Dad. Ruth even showed her the pedal extenders she uses so that she can reach the gas and the brake. Later, Ruth adopted a dwarf boy from Latvia, Janis, who is almost exactly Becky's age and with whom she has become fast friends. (Janis, which is Latvian for "John," is pronounced YAH-nis. His nickname, Jani, is the equivalent of "Johnny," and is pronounced YAH-nee.)

Ruth Ellen Ricker is a remarkable woman whose life parallels the cultural changes in how dwarfism is seen: from a devastating birth defect to an identity, even a source of pride. Born in Calais, Maine, a tiny town on the New Brunswick border, she was the second child and first daughter of George and Wendy Ricker.

George was a struggling young schoolteacher; Wendy, a psychologist, was at that time a stay-at-home mom. In those days little was known about achondroplasia, and the Rickers couldn't believe their daughter would be able to lead a normal life. A bone specialist once tried to cheer them up by saying that Ruth was probably of normal intelligence and could possibly live to the ripe old age of twenty-five or thirty. But a funny thing happened: Ruth thrived. The Rickers moved to a small town just outside of Portland, in part to be closer to Boston, where Ruth's specialists were. Ruth was smart and, aside from ear infections, healthy. Still, they weren't quite ready to trust what they were seeing.

When Ruth was six, the Rickers learned that Little Oscar, the Oscar Mayer mascot and one of the original Munchkins from *The Wizard of Oz*, was coming to their hometown IGA supermarket. They brought Ruth to see him, thinking it would be good for her to meet a dwarf adult. Oscar — Meinhardt Raabe — took to Ruth immediately, and he and his late wife, Marie, stayed in touch with her for many years. More important, he put them in touch with Little People of America. Soon they were attending their first meeting, at a member's home in Massachusetts.

"There was a baby there, and other than that I was the only child," Ruth told me. "It was mostly short-statured adults with all different types of dwarfism, some pretty unique-looking. I was aware that I was short, but I didn't see myself as having any unique structures or proportions — which I certainly do, and did even more at six than I do now. I remember thinking, 'These people are nice, but I'm not like that.' I didn't see myself looking like any of them."

But as her self-awareness grew, her attitude changed: LPA quickly became very, very special. "You know, it was like the magic of Christmas or Disneyland — just being with these other people, kids and adults, who were like me," she said. "And the larger the event, the more significant it was. It's somewhat mystical. It's spiritual. It's a closeness that, from my experience, is only akin to relationships that you develop at camp or in any other intense situation where you're thrown in with people that you might have something in common with."

Ruth underwent leg-straightening surgery when she was fifteen, a turning point that transformed her from a kid whose brother, Bill, pushed her around in the "Rickershaw" — a contraption made of tubing and bicycle tires that a former student of George's had welded together — into an independent young woman. She enrolled at Northeastern University, in part because its massive campus was concentrated in a relatively small area, which would allow her to keep her walking to a minimum. But she soon found herself walking everywhere, as much as a mile to her off-campus job and back. She remained active in Little People of America, helping to plan the 1983 national conference, which was held in Boston, and holding a variety of regional and national positions, culminating in the presidency in 1994.

Ricker proved to be a savvy political activist. When she learned that a then-little-known scientist named John Wasmuth was about to announce that he had discovered the genetic mutation responsible for achondroplasia, she got LPA involved and worked with Wasmuth in order to get out the message that genetic screening should not be used to terminate fetuses with dwarfism if they were otherwise healthy. She got LPA more involved in disability-rights issues, including access to ATMs and gas pumps. When I suggested setting up a dwarfism discussion group on the Internet, she gave me all the support I needed, a step that eventually led to the formation of the Dwarfism List, an interactive forum comprising nearly eighteen hundred members, and LPA Online, the organization's website. She talked about reaching out to gay and lesbian little people and about helping the dwarf community with problems such as substance abuse

— problems well-known in society-at-large, but generally whispered about, if mentioned at all, within a culture that has absorbed too well the lesson that in order to succeed they must be better than everyone else.

And then — to my astonishment, and I'm sure to that of others as well — she walked away after one two-year term, saying she needed to build a life for herself outside of LPA.

I first interviewed Ruth in 1994, for a profile I was doing for Northeastern's alumni magazine. Since then, Barbara and I had become so close with Ruth, and Becky with Jani, that it felt weird to do anything so formal as an interview. But during a summer afternoon, after she'd dropped Jani off with her parents for a week in Maine, she stopped by our house for some time with me and my tape recorder. At forty-two, she seemed happy and fulfilled. She'd been a success as a public person and as a professional since her early twenties. Now, finally, she had built a successful private life for herself as well.

By 1996, she explained, she'd decided that more than anything she wanted to adopt a child, and that she wouldn't have the time to do it unless she stepped down as LPA's president. A civil-rights investigator with the U.S. Department of Education, she could offer a good, stable income and home. Because she would be a single parent, she deliberately sought a slightly older child who would be at least somewhat self-sufficient. And through LPA's adoption program, she learned about Janis. Ruth and her mother traveled to Riga, the Latvian capital, in August 1997, when Janis was just one month shy of his sixth birthday. She took him home and three weeks later she put him in kindergarten. Needless to say, the whole experience was traumatic for Janis — and for Ruth, too.

"I learned enough Latvian so that I could explain, 'Mommy is coming back at the end of the school day.' I was working part-time at that point. I took three weeks off before school started, and that was my maternity leave," Ruth told me.

Nor have Ruth and Jani had an easy time of it since. After she got him to Boston, she realized that he'd been suffering from chronic ear infections — hardly a surprise for any kid with dwarfism. That was cleared up, but, later, he was put on Ritalin and then Adderall to help him concentrate, medication he has continued to use off and on. He repeated the third grade. She takes him to the doctor regularly to deal with a kidney problem. And she still doesn't know exactly what type of dwarfism he has: he meets some of the criteria for achondroplasia, but he doesn't look much like a dwarf except for his short stature, which leads her to think that he might have hypochondroplasia instead.

Such challenges notwithstanding, Janis Ricker today is a happy, well-behaved, mostly healthy boy, a blond kid in glasses who seems never to stop running and jumping around. He and Becky have played at our house, and he is the first person Becky looks for at LPA gatherings. They have even talked about marrying, a subject that is surely a good decade-and-a-half premature. But it demonstrates that they're aware of their differences and of the affinity they have for other people with those same differences.

I wouldn't want to bet a week's pay that Michael Janis Ricker and Rebecca Elizabeth Kennedy will ever walk down the aisle together, but who knows? I do know how important it is that Becky sees Ruth as an intelligent, competent adult with a life as full and rewarding as that of any other adult. And that she understands she and Janis can have that kind of life, too.

The last seven years of Becky's life have been unremarkable — which is, after all, everything we'd hoped for. She goes to a regular public school. She's not treated quite the same as everyone else: the handrails on the stairs and the bathroom have been modified to fit her size, and, until she finally gave it up out of self-consciousness, she sat in a special chair that prevented her legs from dangling. She now keeps a stool under her chair. She takes swimming lessons and is learning to play the clarinet. She's good at it, too. I helped get her started, and one of our favorite activities is to play duets, with me on guitar. She volunteers in the children's room at the town library on Tuesday evenings, when Tim and I are at Boy Scout meetings. She's a Girl Scout. She's been to Disney World twice. She loves our cat, Dexter, and loves to watch TV — so much so that we have to set strict limits. She's funny and talkative and a delight to be with. Her life is so normal that when, a few months before Becky's tenth birthday, Barbara had a chance to return to work full-time at the *Salem News* (the paper into which the *Beverly Times* disappeared after a merger and two sales), she was able to accept it without hesitation.

She's got some quirks. She seems more comfortable with adults than with other kids, and she doesn't like to try new things, whether it's food, books, or riding her bicycle without training wheels. Maybe it's because of all that she went through when she was a baby. Maybe it's just her personality. Whatever the case, we know we're living in a golden period, a bubble, a moment when her dwarfism is not nearly as important as it was when she was younger, or will be when she's older. She hasn't been stuck at home without a date yet. She hasn't been turned down for a summer job by a manager who thinks, but doesn't dare say, that she can't reach the counter, can't lift the trays, can't do this, can't do that, can't keep up with the other employees. Her legs are straight, her back doesn't hurt, and she's not begging us to please please please get her that operation she's seen on TV so that she can be tall like everyone else. All of this may come. But not now, not yet.

Nevertheless, her dwarfism has affected her in subtle ways — so subtle that we're only now beginning to figure it out.

Right after Becky's coming-out party in August of 1995, Barbara and her sister, Mary, took off for Disney World, where they spent a week at my in-laws' time-share condo. For Barbara, it was a much-needed chance to decompress. In September, Becky entered preschool, in a so-called integrated class of kids evenly split between those with special needs and those without. It was a wonderful place for Becky. She started the year speaking no more than one or two words at a time. By Christmas she was well on her way, interrupted only by surgery at Mass Eye and Ear to have her adenoids downsized — pretty much standard for kids with achondroplasia.

During Becky's second year in the integrated preschool we began to receive reports of the trouble she had paying attention in class — that she would lose focus, speak out of turn, couldn't follow directions. While the other kids would gather round for story time, Becky might be in another corner of the classroom, looking at picture books. We were concerned, but she'd been through so much, and was still so young, that we were sure it would resolve itself. The following year she was eligible for kindergarten. Since she would have been the youngest child in her class and she still had some significant delays, we sent her to a private preschool, the same one that Tim had gone to when he was younger. With Becky out of the special-needs environment, we didn't hear much that year about her attentional difficulties.

In first grade, though, Becky's inability to focus returned as a steady, frustrating theme. She was evaluated by the school system's special-education staff and given an Individualized Educational Plan, or IEP, a government-mandated set of goals that is drawn up for all special-ed kids. She was taken out of the class-room a few times a week for help with language skills, help she was still receiving in the fourth grade.

Barbara tried to compensate for Becky's classroom deficiencies by putting in many hours helping her with her homework. But she'd squirm when either of us tried to read to her, squirm when she tried to read by herself, squirm when filling out arithmetic worksheets, and make it very clear that she would rather think about anything other than schoolwork.

From first grade on, we were getting subtle pressure to have Becky diagnosed with attention-deficit/hyperactivity disorder (ADHD) and to put her on Ritalin or a similar medication. We resisted. We certainly didn't reject the idea that medication can be useful for some kids. But we thought that there had to be a better way for someone like Becky, whose problems were subtle, who was not misbehaving in class, and who, despite everything, was still managing to do low-average work. We were also concerned about reports that Ritalin could impede growth. We weren't so much worried that she might end up being three-foot-eleven rather than four-foot-one. But if medication affected the growth of the opening in her spinal column, the effect could be devastating.

Yet the more Barbara tried to do, the farther Becky fell behind. Finally, toward the end of the third grade, we had her evaluated by a child psychologist at North Shore Children's Hospital. His diagnosis: ADHD, inattentive type. After assuring us that he would never recommend medication, he proceeded to do exactly that for the next half-hour. Barbara was ready to try anything. I wasn't quite there yet. In reading about ADHD, I came across a term I hadn't heard before: central-auditory-processing disorder, which, to oversimplify, is characterized by the inability of the brain to understand what the ears are hearing. The symptoms seemed to fit Becky better than ADHD, and she had several risk factors for such a disorder, including a long hospital stay as a baby and frequent ear infections.

What we ended up learning was even more surprising. Becky does, indeed, have an auditory-processing disorder, though not a severe one. Far more important is that she has a slight but permanent hearing loss — a loss that is often more than slight during the school year, when she, like many kids, goes from one cold to another, and her ears are frequently congested and occasionally infected.

The full dimension of Becky's hearing problem was detected by Sandra Cleveland, an audiologist at Northeastern University, who is a nationally regarded expert on processing disorders. I'd brought Becky in to be evaluated, only to be told her hearing was so bad that we should see Dr. Cunningham. Becky told me that her hearing was fine, which Barbara and I realized was itself a sign of trouble: if she perceived her hearing as normal that day, then we knew it must be substantially compromised a good part of the time.

Cunningham discovered that fluid had built up once again behind her left eardrum. He surgically inserted a tiny tube to drain it, just the latest of numerous tubes he'd put in over the years. The eardrum of her right ear was slightly perforated, allowing the fluid to drain naturally. Several weeks later, both Cunningham's office and Sandy Cleveland conducted follow-up tests. The verdict: Becky's hearing was within normal range, as it had usually been when tested over the years. But Cleveland explained to me that Becky's hearing was normal *only for an adult.* It wasn't good enough for a child, who lacks an adult's ability to fill in missing information, and who, unlike most adults, must spend long periods of time in classrooms listening to teachers talk. Cleveland said that Becky could hear if she worked really hard at it, but the effort would become exhausting and, after a while, she'd simply stop paying attention.

Barbara and I were angry with ourselves. For years we had treated Becky as though she had a hearing problem, getting in her face, speaking loudly and slowly. She'd always used some words inappropriately, and occasionally would ask us what, say, *msfnglixzy* means. We'd ask her to repeat it over and over, and it would keep coming out the same way, like she hadn't heard it properly in the first place. But we'd told ourselves that it must be something else, since her hearing had been tested many times over the years and she'd always passed. Cleveland also explained that Becky's diagnosis involved some new thinking as well — that as recently as five or ten years earlier, her level of hearing loss would have been thought by most experts to be harmless. Indeed, Cunningham didn't think Becky's hearing loss was as significant as Cleveland did, a reflection of the difference between their roles: an ear-nose-and-throat surgeon versus a childhood-hearing specialist.

Still, there was something disconcerting about the knowledge that we'd blown it — that despite all we knew about dwarfism, that despite how hard we'd worked with Becky and her teachers in trying to keep her up to speed in school, we'd gone years without realizing that *she couldn't hear.* At least not as well as she needed to.

At the beginning of the fourth grade I met with Becky's teacher, Kathy Picone, and explained to her that her hearing might be off and that we were having her evaluated for an auditory-processing disorder. The results were encouraging. Becky was put right in front, where she could see Mrs. Picone's face and hear her without having to strain. Becky is having her best year so far — not perfect, but a huge improvement over her first three years, when she and other kids would be seated around circular tables and would be expected to listen to the teacher even if their back was to her.

At some point we may need to consider an electronic amplification system to boost the sound of the teacher's voice or possibly even hearing aids, combined with some therapy for her auditory-processing problems.

In retrospect, it all makes sense. When Becky first landed in Mass General, her ears were filled with fluid, yet she was so tiny that Dr. Cunningham couldn't give her tubes. The fluid stayed there for more than a year before he could perform surgery, the pressure all the while building up behind her eardrums. The only reason she avoided a massive ear infection was that she was given antibiotics as a preventative until Cunningham could operate. No doubt her hearing never fully recovered from that experience. Yet we never figured it out.

For me, the lesson is that when you have a child with a disability, you can't stop learning, asking questions, or pushing for more and better answers. Becky could very well have started the fourth grade taking Ritalin. And I have no doubt that we would have been impressed by the results. After all, Ritalin is a performance-enhancing drug that helps sharpen anyone's concentration, regardless of whether ADHD symptoms are present or not. But given that Becky turns out not to have classic ADHD, that doesn't mean it would have been the right thing to do. Her underlying problem would have been masked, not addressed.

We had thought that Becky's learning disability had nothing to do with her dwarfism. In fact, it turned out to explain everything. Because of her dwarfism, her eustachian tubes are tiny and do not drain properly. That poor drainage took a slight but permanent toll on her hearing. I have actually seen Internet posts suggesting that there is at least anecdotal evidence of a link between achondroplasia and ADHD. After our long struggle to figure out why Becky couldn't pay attention, I now wonder whether the real link is between achondroplasia and hearing loss.

This much we know: If we hadn't take charge, we never would have learned the truth. As Becky enters her teens and heads toward adulthood, she'll need to learn how to act as her own best advocate. For now, and for the immediate future, that job remains ours.

Chapter Eleven

Of Drunks and Divas

Using any measure you like, Anthony Soares is a success. By day he's the art director at a Manhattan advertising agency whose clients include AT&T and Philip Morris. In the evenings and on weekends he's the president of the city council in Hoboken, New Jersey, the suburban city where he's lived since buying a condo there in 1991.

On a record-hot April evening, he pulled up in front of City Hall, where I'd been waiting, and waved for me to get in. The night before, I'd watched him preside over the council, attempting to reason with such characters as an elderly woman whose hobby is to show up at meetings and blurt out non sequiturs disguised as questions and a fellow councilor who was so enraged by Soares's unwillingness to derail a housing development that he bellowed, "You're a jerk! You're a jerk!" as soon as the closing gavel had sounded. Soares, an achondroplastic dwarf who was some two feet shorter than his adversary, smiled and walked away. Indeed, on that particular evening he was a picture of tranquility. But it's not always thus. Tom Jennemann, who writes for the weekly *Hoboken Reporter*, told me, "He's very outspoken. He's very, *very* outspoken." Another observer, who refused to identify himself, added, "I've known Tony for a long time. I'm not going to talk about him. My diplomatic instincts intervene here."

I'd seen the two sides of Tony Soares on the Dwarfism List, where he'd made a reputation as an intelligent, articulate, persistent, and angry — very, *very* angry, to paraphrase Jennemann — critic of dwarf entertainers who conduct themselves in what he sees as demeaning, degrading ways. In the mid-1990s he served a stint as Little People of America's vice president of public relations. Among other things, he used his post to speak out against Steve Vento, a dwarf who worked at a Mexican restaurant in Milwaukee by serving chips and salsa from a sombrero on his head. Soares's stand was controversial within LPA — supported by some, but criticized by those with careers in the entertainment business, some of whom have occasionally had to make the same sort of unpalatable choice that Vento made. So when I got into Soares's car that evening, I wanted a chance to talk with him, face to face, about why a person with dwarfism who had achieved such mainstream success would be so exercised over what other dwarfs choose to do with *their* lives.

We drove up and down Washington Street, Hoboken's main drag, Soares's feet working the pedal extenders as he searched for a parking place. Finally he found a spot near an outdoor bistro, where he ordered a beef dish that looked rare enough to get up and walk away. He had a lot on his mind — not only work and city politics, but his health, too. His back was aching, and he'd just returned from Johns Hopkins, where Dr. Michael Ain had examined him. But he was polite and friendly and, yes, outspoken during our conversation, a conversation that was interrupted repeatedly by constituents who approached him to exchange pleasantries and shoot the breeze.

I asked him about something Bill Cosby once said in an interview. I've long since misplaced Cosby's exact words, but, essentially, he complained that excessive concerns about dignity and respect had shut African-American actors out from certain comic roles — that they couldn't be clowns, for instance, without being criticized for embracing negative racial stereotypes. Why, Cosby asked, shouldn't black entertainers have the same opportunity as whites to engage in goofy, physical humor? I asked Soares if he didn't see a parallel between Cosby's critique and the right of dwarf entertainers to make fools of themselves.

"There's a big difference between him acting silly and stupid, and him acting like Stepin Fetchit," Soares replied. "I think there's a big difference between the guy who plays J.J. on *Good Times* and the woman who played one of the space crew in the sixties on *Star Trek*." Then again, Nichelle Nichols, the African-American actress who portrayed Lieutenant Uhura on *Star Trek*, was cast in a dead-serious role, exactly the sort of politically correct part to which Cosby had argued blacks should *not* be restricted. But I let it go. I was more interested in learning why Soares believed dwarfs such as Nacho Man could harm someone like him, an accomplished thirty-eight-year-old professional who hopes someday to be elected the mayor of his adopted city.

Soares told me a story. One morning he was walking his dog when he ran into another dwarf man who lives in Hoboken. While they were talking, a white limousine pulled up, and out jumped a beefy guy who looked like a bouncer, followed by a dwarf. The bouncer — a talent manager, actually — approached Soares and his friend. It turned out that the other dwarf was there for some sort of alleged entertainment event at a Hoboken bar that night, and his manager wanted to know if Soares and his friend would like to make a few extra bucks.

"I think it's horrific what you do to this man," Soares told him by way of reply. "I think this is in poor taste."

"Aw, come on, what else is he going to do?" the manager asked.

"What else is he going to do? Do you assume that I'm some sort of freak?" They were standing outside of Soares's condo. Soares pointed to it and continued, "I live in this building. I own an apartment here." He gestured to his friend. "This man is married, he's planning a family. We're real people."

The manager's response: "Oh, come on. You're a rare case."

"Rare?" retorted Soares. "Get the hell out of this town, buddy." The manager began cursing, and Soares told him, "In another second, I'll have the police here. I'm the president of the city council. You can't come into this town and do this kind of exploitative crap. It's barbaric."

Soares told me there was a lesson in that encounter. "Why do people laugh at little people?" he asked. "The entertainment business. People do not laugh at people going by in wheelchairs, or burn victims. They laugh at dwarfs because it's been made to be okay. They were court jesters, freak-show performers, circus acts, and cute little munchkins with funny voices. It's an automatic response. I can walk down the street and know, based on who I am approaching, that I'm going to get some shit. I can almost sense it."

He added of his happenstance encounter with the dwarf entertainer and his obnoxious manager: "I made a call to the mayor right away, because this guy was harassing me, just as a regular citizen. But they did not stop me because they thought I was just like anybody else. I could have been in a three-piece suit and had on a $10,000 Rolex watch and they *still* would have done that. Because all they saw was *dwarf*. They didn't see anything other than that."

Tony Soares is arguing for group responsibility, for each member of the LP community to carry himself or herself with a certain degree of dignity so as not to contribute to negative stereotypes. "It's almost like empirical data. If you act like a jerk, some other dwarf is going to be hurt by it," he said. It was hard to disagree. He put forth a strong case for why a dwarf who makes a living by making a fool of himself can have a harmful effect on other dwarfs. Yet, personally, I have a hard time accepting the notion that person *X* shouldn't do *Y* because it might make a few yahoos laugh at person *Z*.

Partly this is because of my belief in individual freedom. I'm against rules that ban what another person chooses to do as long as it doesn't harm anyone else — whether it be smoking pot, engaging in exotic but consensual sexual activities, or serving chips and salsa from the top of one's head. But partly — maybe mostly — it's because I've never seen my daughter as being limited in any way by the culture into which she was born. I've always believed that Becky can do anything she wants, as long as she's not looking for a career as a professional basketball player. I can't imagine that what another person chooses to do will have a negative effect on her. Yet Soares's experience suggests that it's not that simple.

Take what happened to Doyle Harris, a dispatcher at the University of Louisville and a former district director of Little People of America. Nearly twenty years ago, he and some friends were waiting outside a Louisville nightclub. It was right around the time that dwarf-tossing — an Australian import that rears its ugly head wherever drunk, stupid men in their twenties gather — had first come to the attention of the media. "One of these guys came out — he was a little inebriated — and he went, 'Oh, they're going to have dwarf-tossing tonight. Well, let me practice,'" Harris recalled. "And the next thing I know, the guy literally picks me up and throws me out onto the grass. It was not a good situation. It was very demeaning to me. I was in fairly nice clothes, I was looking to go out, and I'm out in the grass, rolling around, getting grass stains and muddy. It was totally against my will."

Danny Black, the guy who sells the "Midget Petting Zoo" T-shirts and "magic wands," also works as an entertainment agent and has helped some folks find work at dwarf-tossing events. When I asked him to defend the practice, he told me, "The person who's putting himself most at risk is the same person who's agreeing to be the tossee. It's their equipment, it's their rules and limitations, typically, that set the parameters for how that's run. Who am I to deny you the opportunity to be a news reporter? Who are you to deny the lady at the front desk the chance to be a front-desk clerk? Who are you to deny the lady down the street from being a stripper?"

Black's comments sounded logical enough, and ordinarily I would agree. But Doyle Harris was humiliated — and could have been seriously injured — because of what *other* dwarfs chose to do. Some states, including Florida and New York, have actually banned dwarf-tossing. A dwarf's quest to overturn the Florida law in the spring of 2002 became the subject of a characteristically simplistic commentary by libertarian extremist John Stossel on ABC News's *20/20*. Defending the ban were veteran Little People of America activists Robert and Angela Van Etten, whom Stossel portrayed as a couple of uptight moralists. And yes, I'm uncomfortable with the notion of an out-and-out ban. But I'm even more uncomfortable with what happened to Harris.

Here's another example of how difficult it can be to find the right balance between group responsibility and individual freedom. Feminists and religious conservatives have argued for years that hardcore pornography should be banned on the grounds that it exploits and demeans women. It's an argument I reject on free-speech grounds. Recently, though, I rented a movie starring Bridget Powerz — a.k.a. Bridget the Midget — called *Midget in a Suitcase*. Powerz, a dwarf woman, is literally dragged around in a suitcase — and dropped downstairs, and plopped roughly on beds and couches — only to pop out with a smile on her face, ready for action, whenever the average-size man who possesses the suitcase opens it up. As soon as he's done, it's back in the suitcase and on to the next customer.

Dwarf porn stars are invariably described as "midgets," even though every one whose photo I've found on the Internet, male and female, is in fact a disproportionate dwarf. In other words, even if *midget* were an acceptable word, these performers don't fit the definition. Bridget Powerz is apparently pseudoachondroplastic. Gidget the Midget, another porn star, appears to be achondroplastic. But why describe them accurately when a hateful, dismissive word can be used instead?

And what, precisely, is the appeal of midget porn? Bridget Powerz is a reasonably attractive woman. But it's interesting — and disturbing — to note that even with her tongue stud, her pierced nipple, and her tattoos, she easily could pass for sixteen. Bridget is more popular than Gidget. Maybe it's because she's prettier. Maybe it's because Bridget has been on Howard Stern's show and Gidget hasn't. But maybe — and I suspect this is the real reason — it's because Gidget, with her older face and voluptuous figure, appears to be exactly what she is: an adult woman who happens to be a dwarf. Bridget, by contrast, feeds some sick and dangerous fantasies about sex and children.

I guess it all depends on your personal perspective. To me, Tony Soares's and Doyle Harris's scenarios are abstract, theoretical, not a real threat to my daughter. I can listen to them, process what they have to say, even change my mind about the proper balance between group responsibility and individual freedom. Still, I don't feel it viscerally. With Bridget, I do. And I'm leery of a culture whose attitudes about girls and young women with dwarfism have been shaped — no matter how slightly — by the movies of Bridget Powerz.

These days Bridget is said to be retired from the pornography business, and is trying to launch a new career as a singer. Good for her. Unfortunately for me, unfortunately for my daughter, you can still rent *Midget in a Suitcase* at your friendly neighborhood porno shop. No, I wouldn't ban it. But I wouldn't want Becky anywhere near someone who had rented it and who liked it for all the wrong reasons.

It was only with some difficulty that I was able to arrange an interview with Meredith Eaton. She and her husband, Michael Gilden, a stockbroker and actor, had been burned by a journalist a few years earlier, and that was *before* she'd become a television star. It took the intervention of a mutual acquaintance, a stream of e-mails, and some importuning in the hotel lobby at the 2002 Little People of America conference in Salt Lake City to get her to spend an hour with me. Michael was not with her; she said it was because he was playing boccie — Italian bowling, a staple at LPA gatherings. No doubt he was. But I also suspect he'd made sure he'd *found* something else to do rather than put his trust in another writer. (Note: Their marriage came to a heartbreaking end in December 2006, when Michael Gilden committed suicide.)

Normally I am not particularly flustered by the idea of being in the presence of a celebrity, but there was something about Eaton, looking casually glamorous in a black-and-white ensemble, that threw me. Just as we were about to begin, I realized I'd misplaced my notebook, which left me sputtering incoherently for a moment or two. She reminded me that I'd left it downstairs and waited patiently while I retrieved it.

From *The Wizard of Oz* to the *Austin Powers* movies, dwarf entertainers have been cast as lesser beings, as clowns, as antic window dressing. It can be a pretty discouraging way to make a living. Armistead Maupin's 1992 novel, *Maybe the Moon*, was about a dwarf actress who was the unacknowledged, down-on-her-luck star of an *E.T.*-like movie whose dream was to attain mainstream recognition and success. *Maybe the Moon* was, in fact, loosely based on the life of the late Tamara De Treaux, who really was one of the dwarf performers who donned the E.T. costume and who spent the rest of her career appearing in rubber suits or popping out of refrigerators in forgettable comedies such as *Ghoulies* and *Earth Girls Are Easy*. Of course, *E.T.*, *The Wizard of Oz*, and *Goldmember* aren't *Midget in a Suitcase*, and there's nothing really wrong with dwarf entertainers' making a living by taking advantage of their difference. But Meredith Eaton represents a significant step forward, one that would have been unimaginable even ten years ago: a dwarf actress who plays mainstream characters.

Twenty-seven years old when we met, Eaton told me that she had been accepted into the Ph.D. program in psychology at Adelphi University when, on a whim, she tried out for a role in a movie called *Unconditional Love*, which at this writing was scheduled to be released in the summer of 2003. She got the part, which she describes as that of a strong woman whose dwarfism is incidental. She liked the experience so much that she decided to pursue an acting career and dropped out of school. Which did not, she admitted, make her parents happy.

But Eaton stuck with it and has managed to find work in one non-stereotypical role after another. She played a prostitute in an episode of *NYPD Blue* — a part she accepted, she said, only after the show's creator, Steven Bochco, agreed to tone down the use of the word *midget*. "In the script, the cop says to me — he's referring to one of my prostitute friends — and he says, 'Is Brenda a midget too?' And my famous line that I created is, 'It's *little person*, asshole,'" Eaton told me, laughing in delight. She also played an oral surgeon on an episode of *Dharma & Greg* and was a murder suspect on the *CSI* episode that I referred to in an earlier chapter. (Michael Gilden, by the way, played the victim. At least it wasn't his real-life wife who killed him.)

Eaton may be best known for playing the lawyer Emily Resnick on the now-canceled CBS dramatic series *Family Law*, a role that featured, among other things, a romance between her and a dwarf man, also played by her husband. And her fan mail has convinced her that she's been able to make a difference in people's lives. "I've gotten,

'Thank God, finally, you've played a lawyer, my daughter's being taken more seriously,'" Eaton said. "A woman came up to me and said, 'You know what? I'm respected more in my workplace now. Thank you, thank you for giving me confidence.' So I know I've made an impact in a positive way."

Eaton, who is four-foot-two, has pseudoachondroplasia, like her mother, a psychoanalyst. Her father, who is average-size, is a judge. As a teenager, Eaton said, she went out with average-size boys exclusively; her husband, whom she met at an LPA conference following months of get-acquainted e-mails, is the first little person she had ever dated. Yet her dwarfism has hardly been incidental to her life. Pseudoachondroplasia often carries with it significant orthopedic complications. Eaton told me she'd had sixteen surgeries, mainly to straighten her severely bowed legs. One particularly painful procedure involved drilling holes in her legs and putting on Ilizarov fixators, the same devices that are used for limb-lengthening but which are sometimes used for straightening instead. It didn't work. The fixators had to be removed, and she then underwent another series of operations to straighten her legs by more conventional means.

But despite the impact that her dwarfism has had on her, she suspects that she's been able to act as such a positive role model because her parents told her that it was the least important aspect of her identity.

"My parents always taught me, 'Meredith, you are a person of short stature, you're not a short-statured person,'" she said. "'You are a person first. You are a woman, you are a brunette, you are a daughter, you are Jewish, you are intelligent, you are compassionate. You are this, you are this, you are this, you are this, and guess what? You're short.' That is so important. Now I realize it. At eight, nine, and ten I never understood why that verbiage meant so much. And now I understand why."

The last time I was in touch with her, she sent me an e-mail telling me that she was now trying her hand at screenwriting. "I figure if I want positive, well-developed roles," she said, "I might as well create some!"

A more non-mainstream type of mainstreaming, if you will, can be seen in the 2002 movie *Cherish*, whose stars include Ricardo Gil, a photographer and artist who lives in San Francisco. Gil plays the gay, Jewish, wheelchair-using downstairs neighbor of a woman who has been falsely accused in the death of a cop, and who is confined by an electronic ankle bracelet to a police-issued apartment in a dangerous neighborhood. (In real life Gil, who has a type of dwarfism called cartilage-hair hypoplasia, is ambulatory and married to an achondroplastic woman named Meg. They are the parents of an average-size daughter, Lily.) What's unusual about the part is that there was really no need for it to be filled by a dwarf. The director and writer, Finn Taylor, had created the role for a friend of his, a new-media innovator named Gary Brickman, who was indeed a gay, Jewish, wheelchair-using dwarf. But Brickman died before filming could begin.

Gil had retired from the film business after breaking his neck in a stunt in the mid-1980s, an accident that nearly left him paralyzed and that required two operations to repair. He was forty-five years old at the time that I interviewed him, bearded, and getting around with the help of a cane. I asked him how he got his role in *Cherish*. He explained that he was making his daily visit to the coffee shop at the French Hotel, in Berkeley, when Finn Taylor walked in, noticed him, and invited him to read for the part. Taylor told Gil that a dwarf actor who'd tried out in LA had done fine but for some reason wasn't quite right. Later, Gil learned that he was competing with his brother, Arturo Gil, a full-time actor who has appeared on *Ally McBeal* and who these days is a regular on *The Man Show*. Ricardo said he felt some trepidation after beating his brother out, but added that Arturo remained supportive.

Gil appreciates what a step forward his part was, but he refuses to criticize dwarf actors who have been forced to take stereotyped roles. "I guess we see so many roles that aren't real — fantasy-type characters — and not enough of the character roles that Meredith Eaton did, or that Art did on *Ally McBeal*," Gil told me. "Those are the kinds of roles that I want to see more of. But it's hard for me to say anything against people who are earning a living at being a clown or taking demeaning roles. I've actually taken on some demeaning roles. And the only thing I can do now is possibly take on a role like *Cherish* and show people what a wonderful role this is, and what an interesting role, and promote it, talk about it. I can't be judgmental."

Cherish disappeared almost as soon as it was released, which is a shame. Gil is terrific, a vibrant, foul-mouthed revelation. He told me that he'd written to several reviewers who'd sneered that the only reason Taylor included such an off-the-wall character was to get *Cherish* onto the art-house circuit, not realizing that the part had been intended for Taylor's friend Brickman.

"I didn't blast them," Gil said, "but I told them that the part had been written for his best friend, and his best friend happened to be this, which is fine. And I think I did a damn good job, and you should've mentioned my name in your goddamn review."

The movie may have been something of a commercial flop, but it revived Gil's acting career. For several months afterward he performed eight times a week in the Puccini opera *La Bohème*, which had an extended run in San Francisco before moving to Broadway. Under the direction of Baz Luhrmann — best known for the 2001 movie *Moulin Rouge!* — *La Bohème* was re-imagined as a 1950s-era greaser epic, with Gil as a pimp (a non-singing role) who's protected by a seven-foot-tall bodyguard.

Gil's real passion, though, is his photography, which can be seen on his website, www.ricardogil.com. Much of his work consists of seeing the world from a dwarf's-eye perspective — holding his camera at what is, for average-size people, waist-high, and making the viewer see what *he* sees. His pictures, he told me, are intended primarily for his daughter. A few years ago, a Discovery Channel documentary portrayed his photography as a work of anger, his chance to get even with a world that didn't accept him as he was. "That was a misperception," he said. "I don't know how they slanted it that way." He added: "The resulting piece is good in that it's doing some social activism. The problem with it is that they distorted my story. I wasn't angry. I was in love with my daughter, I was in love with my family. And I thought it was significant and important to document my family, not just for myself, but for my daughter, as a legacy to her, so that when we're old and she's a grown woman, she can look back at these photographs and come to a different understanding than when she was a child."

Even so, Gil must relish the chance to show the average-size majority how he sees *them*, given their refusal to look honestly at *him*. "I've had people practically jump out of their shoes when I come around the corner and they see me," he said. "We're perceived as not being human, like the gnome or the troll under the bridge. We're not treated as regular people, with the same human faults and dilemmas as everyone else. People freak out. There's a frightened look, and uncomfortable laughing. As a little person I just want to shake that person and say, 'What the hell is going on for you? What have you learned? Why do you treat me like this?'"

The answer, I suppose, is that they've been *conditioned* to treat him like that. That will change when more of us come to realize that a lawyer can look like Meredith Eaton. Or that the neighbor downstairs can look like Ricardo Gil. For decades, the entertainment media have taken away. Now, maybe, they're starting to give back.

On Tuesday, September 4, 2001, precisely one week before the world as we knew it came to an end, a thirty-nine-year-old man named Henry J. Nasiff Jr. died in his hometown of Fall River, Massachusetts. The causes of death were reportedly advanced alcoholism and a seizure disorder, complicated by a genetic condition.

If you'd ever heard of Nasiff, it was, no doubt, by his stage moniker: Hank the Angry, Drunken Dwarf. Nasiff was one of a parade of weirdoes, misfits, and pathetic losers who regularly make their way through the New York studios of *The Howard Stern Show*. Known collectively as the Wack Pack, they go by such charming appellations as Gary the Retard, Crackhead Bob, and Beetlejuice, an African-American dwarf who, as a comedic bonus, portrays himself as being mentally deficient.

Nasiff's genetic condition was achondroplasia. His shtick was to show up on the set drunk or pretending to be drunk (most likely the former, since his alcoholism was apparently real enough) and make an obnoxious fool of himself, mouthing such pleasantries as "Go have sex with Jesus Christ, you faggot!" and "I'm not a midget, I'm a dwarf, you asshole!" His objection to the M-word might be construed as Nasiff's sole attempt at self-respect. Needless to say, such a lesson coming from Nasiff was painfully ironic. He had already turned himself into such a freak that P. T. Barnum would have looked away.

When I learned that Nasiff had died, I can't say I was particularly upset. I didn't know him, after all, and his death was not imbued with the sort of sad, tragic circumstances that impels one's heart to go out to strangers. But I learned that Nasiff's life was more complicated, and more closely intertwined with ours, than I would have believed.

The positive image of dwarfism that we want for Becky is about as far removed from the repulsive antics of Hank the Angry, Drunken Dwarf as one can imagine. Yet it seems that, at least on some level, Henry Nasiff desperately wanted to be part of the same community as our daughter. His death notice in the Fall River *Herald News*, to my surprise, asked that donations in his name be made either to Little People of America or the Billy Barty Foundation. And that's not all. I learned from LPA's executive office that, the previous year, Nasiff had paid three hundred dollars for a life membership. Even more surprising, I learned that Ruth Ricker actually knew Nasiff.

"He adored Billy Barty," she wrote in a message to the Dwarfism List. "He called Billy occasionally on the phone ...as he did me. Billy talked to him and seemed to be encouraging him in a positive, mentoring way. I heard from Hank less and less, which I didn't regret honestly, as he got involved in the Howard Stern stuff and his alcohol abuse got even worse. It's sad that his life turned out this way and ended so young. I feel for his parents and his siblings."

Finding all this out didn't exactly make me feel guilty. After all, I hadn't been *pleased* to learn of his death. Like Bridget Powerz or Steve "Nacho Man" Vento, Nasiff certainly had a right to make a living any way he wanted, just as I had a right to pay no attention to him. But among the dwarf community, his behavior was like a dull toothache: always there to be railed against on the Dwarfism List, along with limb-lengthening and the M-word. He was an embarrassment. Toward the end of his life, he may well have been the most famous little person in the country, more famous than Michael Ain, more famous than Meredith Eaton. And no one — no dwarf, no parent of a dwarf — wanted to be thought of as having anything even remotely to do with Hank the Dwarf.

So I suppose I was satisfied, in a small sense, that Nasiff would no longer be able to humiliate himself and, by extension, the community of dwarfs and their families to which we belong. But I did feel a little foolish — foolish to realize that what I had thought I understood was more complex, and more tied up in human pain and weakness and yearning, than it appeared on the surface. Who was I to dismiss Henry Nasiff so coldly? I didn't even know him.

Following Nasiff's death, his website, www.hankthedwarf. com, was turned into something of a shrine. Yes, you could still watch streaming videos of a drunken Nasiff spewing invective at the camera, or buy a keychain emblazoned with HANK SAYS: DON'T DRINK & DRIVE. But it also included messages from his so-called fans and an unctuous tribute from his manager.

What drew my eye, though, was a photo of Nasiff at the age of perhaps five or six, holding a phone to his right ear and looking as happy and carefree and full of life and promise as any child. Nasiff may have died a drunken wretch, an object of ridicule. But once he was a little boy who was loved and fussed over, dressed in crisp new clothes, and photographed so his parents could admire him and show him off to family and friends.

It makes me sick, and more than a little scared, to realize that his parents wanted the same things for him that we want for Becky — indeed, for both our children. I don't assume for a moment that Nasiff became an alcoholic because he was a dwarf. Rather, I imagine that he allowed his dwarfism to be exploited because he was an alcoholic, which is a very different thing. We all try to do what is best for our kids, to teach them right from wrong and guide them as well as we can. Ultimately, though, the choices they make, and the demons they fall prey to, are beyond our control. Nasiff's life and death are a testament to what a heartbreaking endeavor parenthood can be.

In a sense, Henry Nasiff was Tony Soares's opposite. Soares has succeeded in mainstream society; Nasiff was a success only to the extent that he could make money by getting people to laugh at him in disgust. Soares takes for granted his status in the dwarf community as well as in the broader culture; Nasiff was on the outside looking in. Soares believes passionately that dwarfs who act the way Nasiff did harm the image of other dwarfs. I have no idea what Nasiff believed, but if he could have stopped acting like — stopped *being* — a foul-mouthed, drunken lout, he might have agreed with Soares. Like

Charles Stratton, Nasiff exploited himself; but because he lacked Stratton's shrewdness and self-control, he was unable to build a life.

Role models are important, and Nasiff was the role model from hell. To the extent that he had a responsibility to other dwarfs, he walked away from that responsibility many times over. But he had individual freedom, too. His inability to use that freedom wisely makes it no less precious, or necessary.

Some people — be it Bridget Powerz, Henry Nasiff, or the human missiles in dwarf-tossing events — may make life more difficult for other people who happen to look like them. The examples set by others, such as Meredith Eaton and Ricardo Gil, may lead to greater acceptance. But I'm not going to lie awake at night thinking about how all this affects my daughter. She is who she is, and she will be who she will be. Helping her become the best person she's capable of is hard enough work without worrying about how other people have chosen to live their lives.

Ultimately, we are responsible only for ourselves.

Chapter Twelve

The New Eugenics

Sometimes I wonder if I'm kidding myself. For the past ten years I've been searching for meaning, uplift, purpose in Becky's dwarfism. But though I have couched my search in the language of such modern ideas as the value of diversity and equal treatment for the disabled, what I'm really up to may turn out to be very old-fashioned indeed. Even as I reject the notion that God metes out dwarfism either as punishment or as some murky sign of his favor, is it possible that I've been pursuing a false god of science, of progress, of reason? The genetic mutation that causes thanataphoric dwarfism is almost identical to the one that causes achondroplasia. With the former, you die shortly after birth; with the latter, you live and thrive and grow. Maybe the truth is that it's all just random. My quest has been rewarding at times, frustrating at other times. But I have begun to realize that, like life itself, this quest is a journey with no destination.

For me, the whole notion of meaning was dealt its most lasting and significant setback at a news conference on July 29, 1994. It was on that day that a group of scientists, led by the geneticist John Wasmuth, announced in the journal *Cell* that they had discovered the mutation that causes achondroplasia. As I noted earlier, Wasmuth — who, tragically, died the following year — recommended that screening be limited to cases in which both the father and mother have achondroplasia and whose baby would thus have a one in four chance of inheriting the mutation from both parents, an invariably fatal condition known as double dominance. Even so, Wasmuth surely knew he had given us a taste of the fruit from the Tree of Knowledge. That knowledge could one day lead to the very disappearance of achondroplasia and other genetic forms of dwarfism, whether it be in five years, fifty years, or five hundred.

Despite this possibility, much of the early debate over the discovery of the achondroplasia mutation had to do with the opposite scenario: whether a dwarf couple might go to extraordinary lengths — including abortion — for the purpose of ensuring that their baby would be a dwarf. I've collected articles from publications such as *Science News* and the *Journal of Medical Ethics* that discuss the implications of such choices. Yet I'm not sure what those articles prove, except that scientific journals, and scientists themselves, are capable at times of being as sensationalistic as tabloid newspapers. Doctors and scientists I've spoken with in the dwarf community say they're not aware of a dwarf couple's ever having decided to terminate a pregnancy rather than become the parents of an average-size child. No, it's not the sort of news that a husband and wife would announce in their hometown newspaper. But if such a thing had ever occurred, the presumption in the dwarfism field is that word would have gotten around.

Still, it could happen, couldn't it? A study undertaken in 2001 of 186 people with achondroplasia showed that 75 percent believed it was "not at all important" or only "somewhat important" that they learn whether their child would be a dwarf or average-size. Yet 2 percent did report that they would consider abortion if they found out their child would not be a dwarf.

As I discovered one afternoon in Salt Lake City, Dave and Becky O'Hara were intensely familiar with that moral dilemma, even though they are most definitely not among the 2 percent. Both are achondroplastic. Becky was twenty-four when I interviewed them and is three feet nine inches tall. Dave was thirty-one and is four-foot-six. They're the parents of an average-size son, Bryan, who at the age of eighteen months was already nearly as tall as his mother. The O'Haras learned that Bryan would be average-size through amniocentesis. That was fine with Dave, even good news, since he knew that his son wouldn't have to experience the sort of dwarfism-related back problems he'd had. But Becky was upset.

"I went through a mourning period. I did," she told me. "Because you grow up thinking that you'll have a little person. That you'll have a little person or a double-dominant. But the average is always just put in the back. Now I notice a lot more people with their average-size kids. But you grew up thinking you'll have an achon kid. And I got scared. How am I going to control this kid? How am I going to carry him?"

I asked if they had ever considered abortion. "Oh, of course not," Becky answered. "Never. I still love this baby. Now I wouldn't change a thing about him."

There was a certain irony in Becky O'Hara's angst. The image that Little People of America has done so much to promote is one of normality, of families just like everybody else, dwarf parents, dwarf kids. She had so thoroughly internalized that image that she couldn't imagine having a child who didn't conform.

The fate of dwarfism is just the tip of this new world, a world of stem cells and cloning, of genetic engineering and designer babies, a world in which every child will fit someone's definition of perfect. *Or else.* The promise and threat of this new science have implications that go far beyond the relatively small community of dwarfs and their families.

Indeed, within the disability-rights movement as a whole there are few issues as emotional, and as hotly debated. Having fought so hard and so long for the accommodations and respect and understanding they need to become full and equal participants in society, people with disabilities now face the prospect of elimination at the hands of people who don't understand that their lives aren't diminished — just different. Critics have referred to prenatal screening and selective abortion as the "new eugenics," whose aim, as it was with eugenics in an earlier time, is to eliminate anyone who is different, to do away with diversity before it can arrive in the form of a new-born child. Leading thinkers such as Adrienne Asch, a professor at Wellesley College, argue that it's morally wrong to use screening and abortion to do away with a whole range of disabilities, such as Down syndrome, hereditary deafness, spina bifida (not a genetic condition but a disability that can often be diagnosed in utero), blindness (Asch's own disability), and the like. She writes:

> As with discrimination more generally, with pre-natal diagnosis, a single trait stands in for the whole, the trait obliterates the whole. With both discrimination and prenatal diagnosis, nobody finds out about the rest. The tests send the message that there's no need to find out about the rest.

But Asch pushes her argument too far. To an extent, she sounds like the spinal-cord-injury activists who criticize Christopher Reeve for working toward a cure. Well, okay, acceptance is the most important goal, and Reeve may in some small way be contributing to the notion that there's something wrong with being paralyzed. But come on, the man just wants to walk again. There's nothing wrong with that.

Asch writes that she opposes "using selective abortion to avoid any traits," whether the case involves an able-bodied couple wishing to terminate a disabled fetus or a deaf or dwarf couple who want a baby with the same disability as they. Yet she also observes that she and other leading critics of selective abortion are actually pro-choice feminists in other contexts. Thus Asch appears to support abortion rights for any woman *except* when the decision is based on whether or not the fetus would be born with a disability.

To read Asch is to encounter a disability consciousness lurching toward extremism. At one point she criticizes not just the decision to abort a fetus that carries a disability, but also to discard "an otherwise implantable embryo" in which a genetically based disability has been found. Elsewhere, she expresses her disapproval of scientific literature that refers to the "risk" of having a child with, say, Down syndrome or spina bifida. The proper terminology, she explains, is "possibility" or "likelihood."

In a sense, Adrienne Asch is the flip side of the ludicrous Princeton University philosopher Peter Singer, who is best known for writing that the parents of a seriously disabled new-born should be able to kill him within the first twenty-eight days of birth. Singer's position may resonate in the case of some infants with heartbreaking, painful disabilities, and in fact the sort of euthanasia he advocates takes place quietly all the time. But his logic strikes most people, including me, as entirely lacking in any moral sense. He begins by writing about fatal conditions such as anencephaly — the absence of a brain — but then discusses at length cases involving Down syndrome and spina bifida. Talk about the slippery slope. It's the difference between decisions being made by families and their doctors on the one hand, and enshrining such decisions in law and social policy on the other. As the journalist Michael Specter once wrote in the *New Yorker*, "Singer has never been afraid to take pure reason and drive it right over a cliff." Asch, by contrast, takes a position that is highly moral but lacking in logic or, for that matter, any real understanding about how the world works.

Dorothy Wertz, a psychiatrist affiliated with the Eunice Kennedy Shriver Center, in Waltham, Massachusetts, spent considerable time and effort in trying to figure out *exactly* how the world works. To answer Adrienne Asch's critique of genetic screening, Dr. Wertz joked that most abortions already take place for genetic reasons: half of the fetus's genes are from a man with whom the woman does not wish to have a baby. From there, it is a short leap to choosing abortion for genetic reasons such as serious illness, not-so-serious illness, or conditions that simply don't match the prospective parents' vision of the perfect child.

I interviewed Wertz on a cold February day in the sunroom of her home on Massachusetts's South Coast. Her husband was dying of lung cancer. She would die a year later. Nevertheless, she cut a flamboyant figure, tall and with a strong physical presence despite her advanced years, wearing a pillbox hat, turquoise earrings, and an enormous silver-and-turquoise necklace that looked heavy enough to weigh her down. I'd met her years earlier when I took part in a study she'd overseen regarding the attitudes that parents of disabled kids hold toward the medical establishment. I liked her forthright, down-to-earth manner. What I didn't like so much was what she had learned about attitudes toward disability — including dwarfism.

In the late 1990s Wertz conducted a study of about two thousand people — 1,084 genetics professionals, 499 primary-care physicians, and 476 patients. One of the disabilities that participants were questioned about was achondroplasia. The results were stunning. Among the genetics professionals, 57 percent would choose abortion if it were detected in utero; among physicians, 29 percent; and among patients, 24 percent.

To bracket this, let me pull out two other findings. The first pertains to Down syndrome, certainly a serious genetic condition, but one not incompatible with a good quality of life. Here the proportion of genetics professionals who would abort was 80 percent; physicians, 62 percent; and patients, 36 percent. The second involves a genetic predisposition to severe obesity, which is not a disability at all, or even destiny. After all, parents can teach their kids to eat properly and lead healthy, active lives. Yet even in this instance, 29 percent of genetics professionals would choose to abort, as well as 13 percent of physicians and 8 percent of patients.

What's frightening about all of this is that we are closer to screening for such conditions on a routine basis than many people realize. Some day — perhaps in a decade, perhaps two or three — it will be possible to lay out a person's entire DNA on a computer chip, all thirty thousand or so genes, and compare that person's DNA to the ideal. Such chips could be generated for early-term fetuses just as easily as for those already born. Once the use of such technology becomes routine, it would cost "mere pennies per test," as Wertz has written, to screen fetuses for thousands of genetic conditions. Including, of course, achondroplasia and several other types of dwarfism.

Wertz's study points to another potential concern. Across the board, her findings show that ordinary people are far less likely to choose abortion than are medical professionals. (To be sure, one in four ordinary couples would choose abortion if they learned their child would have achondroplasia, which is high by any measure.) Yet it is medical professionals who will counsel couples when they learn that the child they are expecting would have a disability. What kind of pressure will these professionals use to obtain what is, to some of them, the preferable result? If we had learned the fetus Barbara was carrying in the early spring of 1992 would have severe respiratory problems and could have a whole host of other complications as well, what would we have chosen to do? There was no Becky at that point, only a possibility. And the possibility would have sounded more frightening than hopeful.

Little People of America has long argued that prospective parents who learn that their child will have a type of dwarfism should be provided with information about the good lives that most dwarfs lead, and even be given a chance to meet dwarf children and adults. It's a great idea. But will it happen? And at a time of skyrocketing medical costs, are there too many social pressures *against* that happening? There's no doubt that, in many instances, abortion would be in the best interest of insurance companies. Think of all the money they could save if they refused to cover a fetus that has been diagnosed with a potentially expensive genetic condition. Some parents, of course, would not choose abortion because of their religious or moral beliefs. But what about the vast majority of us — the people who regularly tell pollsters that they're pro-choice, although they may be deeply uncomfortable with abortion personally? Would they be able to resist — would they, should they, even attempt to resist — when faced with the possibility of financial ruin?

And abortion is just one part of this, a crude, archaic approach that will likely fade away with improvements in medical technology — improvements that will raise few of the moral qualms that so divide the culture today. For instance, when you think about it, sex is a really messy, random way of reproducing. Sure, it's fun. But look at all the things that can and do go wrong. In his book *Redesigning Humans*, Gregory Stock argues that in vitro fertilization will someday be seen as the only proper way to have children. "With a little marketing by IVF clinics," he writes, "traditional reproduction may begin to seem antiquated, if not downright irresponsible. One day, people may view sex as essentially recreational, and conception as something best done in the laboratory."

Even average-size couples who wouldn't abort a fetus with achondroplasia would, in all likelihood, choose against implanting an embryo with the mutation. You've got five embryos in that Petri dish over there, and you can only implant one. This one has the genetic mutation for Down syndrome; that one has the mutation for achondroplasia; the other three are mutation-free. All right, Professor Asch, which one do *you* think should be implanted?

And thus we will take another step down the road toward the "new eugenics" — a road that, in Stock's utopian vision, will include artificial chromosomes to include spiffy new designer genes that will protect our descendants from disease, help them to live longer, and make them smarter, better, happier, and just generally imbued with oodles of wonderfulness.

Ultimately Stock posits a world in which we're going to eliminate achondroplasia and hundreds, if not thousands, of other genetic conditions, predispositions, and tendencies. And we're going to do it either by eliminating any individual whose genes we don't like — or we're going to change the genes.

Clair Francomano hunched over a desk in the corner of her office at the National Institutes of Health, in Baltimore, carefully drawing a chart to explain the genetics of dwarfism. Dr. Francomano, a longtime member of LPA's medical-advisory board, was among the scientists who, along with the late John Wasmuth, helped discover the mutation that causes achondroplasia. Her article on how the mutation works was published in the *New England Journal of Medicine* about six months after Wasmuth's article appeared in *Cell.*

Each of our cells has forty-six chromosomes, half from our mothers, half from our fathers. The achondroplasia mutation occurs on the short arm of chromosome 4, in roughly the same region that is responsible for Huntington's chorea. In fact, the achondroplasia discovery was an outgrowth of research into Huntington's. Achondroplasia involves a gene known as fibroblast growth factor receptor 3, or FGFR3. The purpose of FGFR3 is to regulate and, ultimately, to turn off — to shut down — the growth of the skeletal system at the right time in a person's development. Because of the FGFR3 gene, sometime between the ages of fifteen and twenty we stop growing. Without the gene, our bones would keep getting longer and longer.

On the maps that geneticists use, the achondroplasia mutation can be found at location 380. Each location, also known as a codon, consists of three nucleotides, which in turn make up the twenty amino acids that are found in the cells of animals, including humans. (There are four nucleotides, abbreviated as A, C, G, and T. All amino acids, as well as some other substances, are made up of various three-nucleotide combinations.) Normally an amino acid known as glycine (CAG) is produced at codon 380. In achondroplasia, a single nucleotide is different: CAG becomes CGG, which is arginine. Arginine is a more active amino acid than glycine. So in a person with achondroplasia, the FGFR3 gene is too active — in effect, it's stuck in the "on" position — and it slows down and distorts bone growth. The long bones of the arms and legs do not grow nearly as much as they would in an average-size person. The skull develops differently. The opening in the spinal column is smaller than it should be. The person is a dwarf.

"It's operating in a manner that's independent of the usual regulations, I would say," Francomano explained. She added: "We don't understand exactly how this mutation results in the effects that we see. There are a lot of people who have been working on this."

Achondroplasia is just one of four types of dwarfism that have been traced to mutations of the FGFR3 gene, but the only one found at codon 380. The other three are all at codon 650, where, in an average-size person, the amino acid lysine is produced. If, instead of lysine, the amino acid is asparagine, then the person has hypochondroplasia, the mildest of the skeletal forms of dwarfism. If it's methionine, the person has SADDAN, a recently discovered form of dwarfism that's an acronym for "severe achondroplasia with developmental delay and acanthosis nigricans," that last bit referring to skin discoloration that comes with the condition. If it's glutanic acid, then the person has thanataphoric dwarfism, which results in death either at birth or shortly thereafter. One location, three different mutations, ranging from the most benign to the most lethal forms of dwarfism.

By understanding the genetic mutations that underlie dwarfism, it's possible to visualize precisely how it might be treated or even eliminated. But transforming that vision into reality could be extraordinarily difficult. Let's turn our attention back to achondroplasia. With genetic engineering, the middle "G" in CGG at codon 380 would be knocked out and replaced with an "A," and the person literally would not have achondroplasia: she would be "cured" and would in all respects be no different from an average-size person. But for this to work, the change would have to be made in each of the body's billions upon billions of cells, seemingly an impossible task. Francomano told me that performing such a feat at, say, the eight-cell stage, right after a fertilized ovum has developed from zygote to embryo, might be possible; but that presumes in vitro fertilization (IVF). And, as we have already seen, with IVF there is little reason to fix a genetic mutation in an embryo. It's far easier to discard it and implant another embryo instead.

It would seemingly be more practical to treat the effects of the mutation rather than eliminate the mutation itself — to find a way to stop the FGFR3 gene from being hyperactive, to block the effect of the arginine, to get it to behave more like glycine, which would allow the long bones to grow normally and the spinal canal to open up. Here, too, the prospects of developing an effective treatment are daunting. Francomano told me that such a treatment would still have to get around the problem of modifying the behavior of the FGFR3 gene in each of the body's cells.

Francomano is not alone in her skepticism. Among the most experienced dwarfism doctors in the world is Charles Scott, a semi-retired geneticist based at the Alfred I. duPont Hospital for Children, in Wilmington, Delaware. Dr. Scott, who chaired LPA's medical-advisory board from 1969 to 2000, still follows some four hundred patients. I spent a day with him as he made the clinical rounds. Unlike the intense, almost frantic days put in by Michael Ain and Dror Paley, Scott will give an hour or more to each patient, asking questions, listening carefully to the answers, joking, measuring, pulling out an old Polaroid camera to take pictures for his files. Of course, Scott's job is different: he's not a surgeon, and he follows his patients over a period of years rather than through one acute surgical episode. Still, watching him examine kids whose needs range from the minimal (such as Abby Trifone, a nine-year-old achon from Connecticut who's so healthy that she plays lacrosse) to the complicated (such as twelve-year-old Danielle Frank, from Pennsylvania, whose achondroplasia has required several surgeries for spinal compression and who was in a wheelchair when I met her) was to observe someone with unusual empathy and patience.

Like Francomano, Scott was dubious when I asked him about the prospect for treatment either by manipulating the genes or by somehow modifying their behavior. "The actual cure, in my opinion — your great-great-great-grandchildren may benefit from it," he told me. "It's a lot of hype by the feds and the people in research. It's not going to help anyone who has it who's alive today. Not at all. Because the gene is in every cell, and you're made up of ten to the twenty-seventh power. How could you fix a gene in that many cells?"

And yet there remains the fact that people are trying. A few months ago I received a packet of information from the mother of a baby girl with achondroplasia, a mother with a Ph.D. and a scientific background and a dream that her daughter won't have to go through life as a dwarf. The information pertained to an Israeli company, ProChon Biotech, founded in 1997 by a scientist named Avner Yayon.

Among the products that ProChon is working on is a treatment for achondroplasia that will slow down the activity of the FGFR3 gene — that will "prevent or decrease the level of signal transmitted through the receptor," as the company's website (www.prochon.com) puts it. Clinical trials could begin as early as 2003, according to ProChon. Treatment would likely take the form of a drug that would be injected on a regular basis from infancy through adolescence. And despite the skepticism expressed by Dr. Francomano and Dr. Scott, the medication apparently would not have to reach each of the body's cells: according to an e-mail I received from Myriam Golembo, project manager for skeletal genetics at ProChon, the drug would only need to target FGFR3 activity in the growth plates of the bones. "Although definitely not a trivial task," she said, "it is somehow less daunting."

Is this real? Is the end of achondroplasia at hand, at least for those with the money and the ambition to seek treatment? I have to admit that I'm skeptical. American dwarfism specialists whom I interviewed, including Francomano and Scott, were only slightly aware of ProChon. And, as we all know, new medical treatments can have unproven consequences.

The type of dwarfism caused by growth-hormone deficiency, as I noted earlier, has been all but eliminated in the United States through injections of human growth hormone, or hGH. But those who began treatment in the 1960s and 1970s got their hGH from the pituitary glands of cadavers, leading some to develop Creutzfeldt-

Jakob disease, a devastating, fatal brain illness that is similar to mad-cow disease. Today's synthetic hGH is presumably safe. Yet there remain unanswered questions as to whether even synthetic hGH might be associated with a greater likelihood of developing cancer. What once looked like a cure for one type of dwarfism now carries with it unanticipated complications and ethical dilemmas.

Let's say that, when Becky is twelve or thirteen, ProChon's treatment for achondroplasia is determined to be safe and effective. (This is merely hypothetical, since it assumes an unimaginably fast review-and-approval process by the Food and Drug Administration.) I'm not sure she could even benefit at that age, coming so late in her growth. And, naturally, I would worry about side effects that might not crop up for decades. But it would be tempting to try and to give her treatments until her mid- to late teens. I don't much care if she might end up two or three inches taller. But if her spinal canal opened up a little more, if her back straightened out a bit, if her arms grew another inch or so — now those are changes that would give her a healthier, easier, more convenient, more pain-free life.

Little people I've talked with understand this. To a person, they vociferously object to limb-lengthening, yet have no such philosophical problems with the idea of a cure or a genetically based treatment. They see one as torture, as a brutal attempt to make dwarfs fit the human-made environment rather than the other way around. But they see the other as a natural product of scientific research, a medical treatment no different from any other medical treatment.

Daniel Margulies, a past president of Little People of America, already knows what it's like to have seen his form of dwarfism eliminated. Margulies's is a rare case: he got Crohn's disease as a child. Combined with familial shortness, he ended up being four-foot-eight. With today's Crohn's treatments, though, the disease would have affected him to a much lesser extent. He thinks he probably would have been at least as tall as his brothers, who are five-foot-four and five-foot-six.

"I tell people I had to learn to become a dwarf," Margulies said. "Up until I was a sophomore in high school or thereabouts, the doctors told me, 'You will grow. You're going to get a growth spurt.' Finally, they said, 'You're not going to grow. This is your final height, and you need to learn to accept it.' And when the quote-unquote experts have been telling you for years that you're going to grow, and to suddenly be told okay, this is it, learn to deal with it — as a teenager, it's a huge, huge culture shock."

Perhaps because of his personal experience, Margulies understands that more traditional forms of dwarfism may some day be cured as well. "Just as a total lay person who reads the news, I would not be surprised if in thirty years, forty years, if not sooner, somebody's going to say, 'If your child is born an achon, we can now do this, this, and this,' and they will manifest none of the orthopedic structures of an achondroplastic dwarf."

I asked Margulies how popular such a treatment would be. "I would say 95 percent of average-size parents would do this," he replied. "And speaking only for myself and not the organization by any means, I would understand it and see no problem with it. I suspect a large segment of LPA would feel the same way."

But would we be losing something? Would the culture be poorer if dwarfism — or at least the most common form of dwarfism — were eliminated? "Well, my opinion is yes," Margulies said. "You lose diversity, and is diversity good? Yes. Nature has created sex on purpose — half of the genes from each parent, and that creates diversity. Socially, I suspect the same thing. I guess the philosophical question is to what degree is it my responsibility as a parent of a dwarf child to be responsible for that diversity. Why is it put on me? It makes for an interesting philosophical discussion that has no right answer."

And the truth is that if there had been a safe, effective, proven treatment for achondroplasia when Becky was born, Barbara and I would have chosen it without hesitation. How could we not have? I understand and respect dwarf parents who want their own children to be dwarfs. But for the average-size parents of a baby who's just been diagnosed with achondroplasia? Frankly, I suspect Margulies's estimate that 95 percent would seek treatment is approximately 5 percent too low.

Genetic diversity may be what's best for the human race, but giving Becky the gift of health and normality — of a life free of backaches or even paralysis, of respiratory problems, of hearing loss, of orthopedic surgery . . . hell, of discrimination, of being stared at, pointed to, snickered about — well, what parent *wouldn't* do that? The truth is that dwarfism has been a lot better for me than it's been for Becky. After all, I've met a lot of interesting people, broadened my horizons, even got a book contract out of it. I'd like to think it's taught me to be a better, more sensitive person, more attuned to people who are different, and a more caring, patient father. But how, precisely, has dwarfism benefited her?

That's harsh. It may seem like a negation of Becky's place in the dwarf community, as a rebuke to our friends in LPA. I don't think it is. Certainly they, more than I, understand how difficult it can be to live with dwarfism. I would even go so far as to say that I admire their courage, except that — as Benedict Lambert, the brilliant geneticist with achondroplasia who is the lead character of Simon Mawer's novel *Mendel's Dwarf*, puts it — "In order to be brave, you've got to have a choice."

Barbara and I would have chosen not to be brave and not to have forced our daughter to be brave. We would have sought treatment for the effects of Becky's mutated gene just as readily as we would for any other medical condition. Diversity may be a good thing, but, as Daniel Margulies observed, I can't see why the responsibility is ours. Eliminating achondroplasia from the gene pool may have unintended consequences, consequences society will one day regret. But eliminating achondroplasia from the genes of Rebecca Elizabeth Kennedy, or somehow countering the effects of her overactive FGFR3 gene, would have been an entirely good thing.

In the decades to come, such dilemmas will only multiply. Any mother, for instance, would choose to fix her child's genetic predisposition for bipolar disorder, or manic depression, as it used to be called. It's a devastating mental illness. Yet if you took away Robert Schumann's manic depression, he might not have been a musical genius. A non-bipolar Abbie Hoffman might be a living but unknown college professor instead of a dead, wildly creative political iconoclast. Or consider homosexuality, which scientists today regard not as an illness at all but, rather, a normal part of human variation. If a genetic proclivity for same-sex attraction is ever discovered, and indeed there are researchers looking for such a variation, then many parents may opt to edit out that trait as well. Some may do it out of fear or prejudice, but others may simply believe that life as a lesbian or as a gay man is just too hard. Who doesn't want to make life easier for their kids? But what will we have lost?

I've come to realize that my quest for meaning — my goal of attaching some larger significance to Becky's dwarfism — is every bit as limited by my cultural preconceptions and the era in which I live as those who, in decades past, thought that disability was a sign of God's displeasure. The quest is worthwhile, but the destination keeps receding, even as I keep moving toward it.

What's truly meaningful is to be the best parent you can be.

Chapter Thirteen

A Place of Her Own

The dancing begins every night at nine. There's nothing unusual about the scene: lots of gyrating, lots of strategically exposed female flesh, lots of furtive and not-so-furtive attempts to hook up for a night, a week, forever, whatever. But I see trouble. Big trouble.

You see, this particular dance is taking place at the 2002 annual conference of Little People of America. I'm looking right past the teenagers and twentysomethings who are shimmying the night away at the Marriott Downtown in Salt Lake City. Instead, I'm looking into the future. And I'm as ambivalent about what I'm seeing as the father of any pre-teenage girl would be. Becky is not with me in Salt Lake; I'm here alone for a week of interviews, listening, and learning. But I have no doubt that, in a few years, she'll be an eager participant in the mating ritual that's playing out in front of me.

Not that there's anything untoward going on. But when you're about four feet tall, as most of these dancers are, with disproportionately short arms and legs, and you don't move as quickly or as gracefully as your average-size friends back home, the LPA dances take on a certain, shall we say, *intensity*.

Many of these young people have traveled to Salt Lake specifically to meet members of the opposite sex who are as short as they are. For some, the conference is a way to jam a year's worth of dating activity into a week. Relationships are formed here, relationships that are sustained by e-mail and outrageous phone bills and, for the fortunate, occasional plane tickets. Marriages between dwarfs often begin at an LPA conference — marriages that can lead to kids and success and happiness forever after. Or to divorce, as they realize, long after the glow has faded, that they have little in common other than being short.

It's all very normal. But so are a father's anxieties.

For a dwarf teenager, the LPA dances are the answer to fifty-one weeks' worth of phones that don't ring, Saturday nights at home, a nonexistent social life. Barbara and I have not yet been the parents of a teenage girl, never mind one with dwarfism, and we are looking forward to it in the same way that we would look forward to, say, dental work: that is, as something to get through and, presumably, survive. Those with more experience than we say the teenage years can be something of a black hole in the life of an LP. When they're younger, they're popular and have plenty of friends. When they're older, if they're mature enough and lucky enough, they start building a life for themselves. But *during* — well, that's another matter.

Teenagers wouldn't be caught dead wearing the wrong jeans or the wrong sneakers. Soon Becky is going to learn what it feels like to be wearing the wrong *body*. What boy wants to go out with the Dwarf Girl, the *Midget*, the one with the big head and the butt that sticks out, who waddles back and forth and only comes up to his waist? Unless, of course, he wants to take advantage of her and snicker to all of his friends about it. And, no, dating isn't necessarily an essential part of high school. I never did much, certainly not as much as I would have liked. Neither did Barbara, who attended an all-girls Catholic school. But to believe you've been excluded because you look different from everyone else must make it much worse. And it's not just dating. Once, during a parents' meeting at an LPA regional conference, we heard from a mother whose daughter's former best friend — a girl — refused to be seen with her now that they had both reached adolescence. It's all about image, and this is the age at which the image of dwarfism changes.

Young kids with dwarfism are cute. Teenagers with dwarfism, like adults, can be attractive or not, fat or thin, agile or stiff. But they're not cute. Rather, they look like a cross between an adult and a child, with a body the size of an eight-year-old's but with muscles and facial hair, or breasts, hips, and acne. And, except when they're home with their own families, they spend most of their time with other teenagers, kids who lie awake at night agonizing that their *noses* are too big, and who — no matter how compassionate they might have been when they were seven, eight, nine years old — suddenly have no tolerance for or understanding of any type of physical difference.

The LPA conference can be an answer to all this. What I worry about is that it can become *the* answer — an anxiety-laden week that, if it fails to measure up to expectations, can be just as heartbreaking as the other fifty-one weeks. Or more heartbreaking, given that this is where it's supposed to be different. It must be devastating for kids who meet rejection during the fifty-second week as well. There's a pecking order within LPA just as there is in society-at-large, and that pecking order favors good-looking, mobile young people with achondroplasia. It's an open secret within LPA that kids who are more disabled, with more exotic forms of dwarfism, can find LPA to be a fairly inhospitable environment.

And there's a flip side, just as worrisome and potentially a lot more dangerous. For some teenagers and young adults, the conference is the one place where they drink as much, show off their bodies as much, and have as much sex as their friends back home. *All in one week.*

As every parent knows, there are many things worse than your child's being home on a Saturday night.

More than thirteen hundred people have showed up in Salt Lake City during Fourth of July week. It appears that roughly half of them are dwarfs, the other half average-size family members. This is my first national conference. We've attended a number of regional conferences, where Becky has practiced her dance moves with her friend Jani Ricker. But this is bigger than any gathering I've seen.

At any time of the day or night, the hotel lobby is swarming with little people. The achons predominate, and, since they tend to be the healthiest, with the fewest disabilities, I often see them walking, running, or just lounging around. The second-largest group comprises those with diastrophic dysplasia, who usually undergo numerous orthopedic surgeries from childhood on; many of the diastrophics zip about on scooters to cut down on the amount of walking they have to do. Those with SED can grow to well over four feet, but some are tiny, just three feet tall or less. There's another group of children here with primordial dwarfism, a very unusual condition with an adult height of well below three feet. And there are many other varieties as well, some that probably have never been properly identified or diagnosed.

Throughout the week, people walk up to me, scrutinize my name tag, and say, "Oh, *you're* Dan Kennedy." My volunteer work with the organization's website, LPA Online, and with the Dwarfism List land me in controversy from time to time, so when these encounters take place I'm sometimes not sure whether to extend my hand or duck. (Of course, in this crowd ducking would just make it easier for someone to punch me in the face.) But the people I meet are remarkably friendly and supportive. A few are surprised to learn that I'm not a dwarf. One person, inexplicably, said he'd expected me to look like Jerry Garcia.

Thus I quickly lost the degree of anonymity with which the Internet had provided me — an anonymity that, in truth, I hadn't really given much thought to. I had come to learn, and I did. What I hadn't expected was that, just by being there, I had given others a chance to learn something about the mysterious figure behind LPA's Internet presence — the "ghost," as the outgoing president, Leroy Bankowski, jokingly put it at one of the sessions.

Such anonymity is something most little people never experience. From childhood on they are known to all, loved, scorned, overindulged, and laughed at. Many LPs have told me that as far back as they can remember, everyone knows their name.

Here in Salt Lake City, for one week, things are different. They can be just like everyone else.

Almost as soon as Becky was well enough to travel for an hour or two, we began attending local LPA functions, sometimes large gatherings at hotels, sometimes small receptions in people's homes. We hosted one ourselves, too. We've been what I would call middling LPA members — more active than some, less active than many, realizing it was important to Becky's future while at the same time being aware that she often found such gatherings "boring," a judgment she has never hesitated to share with us or anyone else within earshot.

So why is involvement important? LPA members themselves, especially the active ones, have often told me that it's absolutely essential for any person with dwarfism, and for their families as well. They speak of the isolation they felt before getting involved — and of the shock they experienced at seeing so many people who looked like them. "I walked in the door and I froze, because I'd never seen so many little people. It was my very first meeting," said Al Staples, a sixty-six-year-old hospital volunteer and retired jeweler who lives in the Boston area. At four-foot-four, Staples said he also experienced something else for the first time: "I was the tallest of all of them." Like many LPA members, Staples met his future wife, Celeste, at a meeting. Celeste Staples, who had a medically complicated type of dwarfism called Morquio syndrome, passed away several years ago, but Al remains an active member.

Still, with roughly four thousand dwarf members and another four thousand average-size family members and friends, LPA reaches only about 10 percent of the dwarf community. Some join, find a mate, and leave. But some obviously either don't need it or don't want it. LPA is not necessarily a representative sample of the dwarf population. For instance, LPA is overwhelmingly white, which may speak to different attitudes about dwarfism in other ethnic groups. Its members — certainly those who can afford to attend national conferences every year — tend to be professional, well-educated, and affluent. Although it's hard to know for sure, the organization's membership base is thought to be disproportionately weighted toward people with achondroplasia, since their relatively good health allows them to be more active. What all this means is that LPA is not *the* dwarf community but, rather, a certain *type* of dwarf community. Above all else, members are the kinds of people who think of themselves as a community, which is not a given, but a predisposition, a state of mind. Not everyone, after all, is a joiner.

When I was in high school, I read Kurt Vonnegut's novel *Cat's Cradle*. I only remember two things about it: "Ice-9," a form of water developed by atomic scientists that freezes at room temperature, and, in the end, destroys the earth; and the made-up word *granfalloon*, which Vonnegut defines as "a proud and meaningless association of human beings." A granfalloon, Vonnegut writes, might consist of people who belong to the same religious organization, or who come from the same state, and who are naïve or foolish enough to believe that those coincidental ties are meaningful. Might LPA be a type of granfalloon? I enjoy belonging to the organization, mainly because

I've met a lot of interesting people I otherwise never would have gotten to know, and because I think it will be important for Becky's future. It's a great place to get information about dwarfism. And, obviously, dwarf members who are looking for a mate the same size as they have few other places to turn. But what, really, do LPA's more than eight thousand members have in common other than being under four-foot-ten — the organization's rough guideline for membership — or being related to someone who is?

I have heard it said that dwarfs who want nothing to do with LPA are in "denial." I'm sure that's true in many cases. Not long after Becky was born, I read an article by a journalist named John Wolin, a middle-aged achondroplastic dwarf who was attending his first national conference. Wolin wrote frankly about his decades of denial, and of the envy he felt for a woman who had agreed to act as his guide: "She was years, a lifetime of self-acceptance, ahead of me." But surely there must be dwarfs who accept themselves and yet who see no need for LPA — or who accept themselves and their genetic condition in ways that the typical LPA member would find abhorrent.

During my visit to Dror Paley and John Herzenberg's limb-lengthening clinic in Baltimore, for instance, none of the dwarf kids and average-size parents whom I interviewed had ever been active in LPA. *Ah, ha!* you might say. They were undergoing painful, risky surgery because they had never accepted themselves or had never been accepted by their parents. But what they told me — what I saw — was that they had accepted themselves in a different way: that they had a genetic condition, a disability, that was hampering their everyday lives. And that they could undergo surgery to lessen the effects of their disability. It was true. That is, it was *a truth* — not the same truth that you'll hear at an LPA conference, but a truth nevertheless.

The sociologist Erving Goffman writes that organizations for stigmatized people tend to denigrate those who share their stigma but who choose not to associate with them. "If he turns to his group, he is loyal and authentic; if he turns away, he is craven and a fool," Goffman says. "Here, surely, is a clear illustration of a basic sociological theme: the nature of an individual, as he himself and we impute it to him, is generated by the nature of his group affiliations." Which is, I suspect, why some LPA members get so worked up when they talk about people who've undergone limb-lengthening. It's not just that they subjected themselves to a potentially dangerous, unnecessary medical procedure. It's that they have rejected their group identity — or, rather, the group identity that LPA says they should have. I understand. But I can see the other side, too.

By embracing LPA and letting LPA embrace us, we have adopted certain truths — not absolute truths, but truths that are comfortable for us. That there is a dwarf community. That being part of it is a good thing. That self-acceptance consists of trying to see the positive as well as the negative aspects of dwarfism. And that a person with dwarfism has a difference, not a disease, and is not someone who is broken and must be fixed.

It is only by imbuing LPA with such meaning that the group avoids becoming a granfalloon and instead becomes a living, breathing, growing organism.

At the LPA conference in Denver, in 1995, the psychologist Len Sawisch gave a presentation on attitudes about dwarfism. He talked about a time that he had visited a dwarf couple whose home had been completely retrofitted to accommodate their height, right down to the shower head. In such an environment, Sawisch asked, can dwarfism truly be said to exist?

"It was amazing," he told the audience. "I was still me. My body was still this body. Was I a dwarf in that context? It really became confusing for me, and yet it became clear for me that dwarfism is not a thing, it is a kind of relationship. It takes on meaning only in the context in which we find ourselves."

In other words, if everyone were between three and four feet tall rather than most people being between five and six feet tall, then there would be no such thing as dwarfs. There would be no doors, coat racks, ATMs, gas pumps, or elevator buttons that would be out of reach. And no one would be suggesting that *they* were the ones who needed to be changed, rather than the constructed environment being changed in order to accommodate them.

Early on during my week in Salt Lake City, I went out to dinner with Robert Van Etten and his wife, Angela Muir Van Etten. Robert, a fifty-two-year-old rehabilitation engineer, is a past president of LPA; he has SED and is three-foot-five. Angela, forty-eight, is a past president of Little People of New Zealand, her native country. She has an exceedingly rare form of dwarfism known as Larsen syndrome and stands three-foot-four. Like many middle-aged people with dwarfism, their mobility is limited but not entirely absent. Robert rode their wheelchair to the restaurant but told Angela that she could ride it back to the hotel.

Both Van Ettens have been heavily involved with access issues over the years — especially Angela, a lawyer who was appointed during Ruth Ricker's presidency of LPA to serve on the so-called ANSI Committee, part of the American National Standards Institute. ANSI is a private organization that drafts model accessibility codes. Its codes are not law but are often adopted by government regulatory agencies. The issue is one that has preoccupied her since her youth. In her autobiography, *Dwarfs Don't Live in Doll Houses*, she writes of the frustration she encountered in law school in New Zealand, where the elevator buttons were just out of reach:

> The law library was on the fifth floor and the lecture rooms were on the sixth. However, the highest button I could reach on the elevator was number four! On the days when I was feeling

energetic, I would walk the extra one or two floors, but that wasn't very often. Otherwise, I would wait for someone to come or use an object such as my pencil case or umbrella to reach the button.

Things are better today, better in the United States than in New Zealand and most other countries, and getting better all the time. But there is still a long way to go. Angela Van Etten told me about her advocacy work during the past decade. It was a long, tangled tale of bureaucracy run amok, but basically what happened was this. When the Americans with Disability Act was signed by the first President Bush, Little People of America was not as involved as it should have been on disability issues, and thus the specific needs of dwarfs were not addressed. Automatic teller machines — ATMs — as well as self-service gasoline pumps were set at no more than fifty-four inches high, which is within the reach of a wheelchair-user with average-size arms but not within the reach of most little people.

LPA undertook a study — actually measuring people at a national conference — and found that forty-eight inches was the maximum height that most dwarfs could reach. After years of agitating, ANSI and the federal government finally went along with a forty-eight-inch height for ATMs, and it is moving in that direction for gas pumps as well. The elevator industry has also proved cooperative, mainly because new computer technology will allow for the installation of just a few buttons on elevators even in very tall buildings, rather than the one-button-per-floor arrangement that is predominant today. The revised standards pertain only to new construction, and it will no doubt take many years before their effects are widely seen. Still, they are a crucial step in the right direction.

"We don't care how you do it," Angela told me, describing the ANSI philosophy. "We don't ask you to lower anything. If you can't lower it for whatever reason, just provide an alternative. It's usability that we're looking for. I've actually said this to them: 'We do not expect the world to get down on its knees.' It's a matter of industry will to recognize this population. They generally will not do it unless you make them."

The concept behind accessibility is something that advocates refer to as "universal design." The idea is to make facilities accessible to the disabled and able-bodied alike, and to do it in such a way that it not only doesn't inconvenience the able-bodied but actually helps them. The classic example is curb cuts, which have turned out to be as much of a godsend for parents pushing strollers as for wheelchair-users.

Cara Egan, a thirty-five-year-old former vice president of public relations for LPA who has achondroplasia, wrote her master's thesis at Johns Hopkins University on LPA's role in public-policy areas such as accessibility. She was so busy in Salt Lake that I didn't have a chance to interview her. But I caught up with her at her home near Washington, D.C., several weeks later. At one point I walked up to an ATM to get some money for the parking garage. It was at a comfortable level for me, but barely reachable for her. She asked, "Would it really have inconvenienced you if the machine had been built maybe a foot lower?" Of course not, I replied.

That led to a discussion of one of the principal arguments for limb-lengthening: that it makes dwarfs more functional in a human-made environment built for people between five and six feet tall. "I think that's bullshit," Egan said, explaining that such a philosophy assumes it's the *person* who should be changed rather than the *environment.* The beauty of universal design, she said, is that it makes things accessible for everyone. "I was able to get down to the Metro today, park my car, put money in the meter, go down and get a Metro fare card, go downtown, and I didn't have to ask anybody for anything," she said. "We have shown that we can do it, so why not do it? We've got the creative energy. I think that's a total cop-out. My mother is five-nine. She goes into the grocery store and there are things that she cannot reach. And she will ask somebody to help her."

Egan does most of her own grocery-shopping at a store in nearby Rockville, Maryland, that has been redesigned with shorter shelves and smaller carts. "And it's not like the tall people are staying away, because it's easier for everybody," she said. "I just think we're getting smarter about how things are designed."

As I learned during my time in Salt Lake, there is a certain ebb and flow to a national conference. Mornings are for meetings — parent receptions, discussion groups for people with particular types of dwarfism, LPA business meetings, and the like. Afternoons are less hectic, as families generally leave to go sightseeing; it turned out to be a good time to conduct interviews. Evenings are for events such as the fashion show and the talent show and, on the last official night, the banquet. The talent show was a particular highlight, especially when Bill Bradford — one of three brothers, along with Randy and Dave, with diastrophic dysplasia, all of them holding top LPA positions — did a comedy routine.

"I have a teenage daughter, which I think is worse than having three diastrophic boys," he said. He told of running into someone who asked, "How long you been short?" His response: "How tall you been dumb?" But the one that brought the house down was about a guy whose pants were hugging his hips and who asked if he could call Bradford "Shorty." His comeback: "You can call me 'Shorty' if I can call you 'Butt Crack.'"

The LPA conference also coincides with the annual games of the Dwarf Athletic Association of America, or DAAA. A lot of younger people were clearing out every morning to take a bus to nearby West High School, where dwarfs were competing in track and field, soccer, swimming, volleyball, and basketball; a boccie tournament was taking place back at the hotel. Normally weightlifting is a big draw, but Pam

Danberg, the president of the DAAA, told me that scheduling problems had forced her to cancel it, as well as table tennis and badminton.

Danberg, a forty-four-year-old achondroplastic dwarf, is herself an accomplished athlete. I've seen photos of her throwing the javelin in several LPA publications. Just before the DAAA games she had been appointed to the President's Council on Fitness and Sports and had been sworn in by President George W. Bush on the White House lawn. She's also on the board of directors of the U.S. Olympic Committee. Her husband, Scott Danberg, who has hypochondroplasia, is a fitness director at a health resort and a star on the Los Angeles Breakers, a dwarf basketball team.

The main purpose of the DAAA, Pam Danberg told me, is to reach out to dwarf kids, who normally have little chance to play sports with their average-size peers. "A lot of kids don't get the same opportunity to compete at home on the same level," she said. "And I try to teach an active lifestyle, especially with an epidemic of obesity in the country. We're a fast-food, no-movement society. I teach socialization, competition, and fair play."

I tried to picture Becky at the DAAA games. As you already know, she's pretty good at miniature golf and candlepin bowling, and she loves to swim and ride her bike, even though she couldn't keep her balance without training wheels until well after her tenth birthday. But she has never expressed any interest in playing sports with kids her own age. She tried boccie at an LPA regional conference, but the waiting around drove her crazy.

Thus unlike Tim, who plays baseball and basketball and who's even made the Little League all-star game as a pitcher, Becky's athletic activity has been pretty much restricted to occasional outings with her parents. Yet we know she needs to be more active and that, given the right context, she'd have a great time. She likes to play catch in the backyard. Once there was a softball clinic at an LPA regional, and she couldn't get enough. Whether it was her love of the game or her excitement that her friend Jani was there didn't really matter. For an afternoon, she was running around like any other kid, something she doesn't do nearly as often as she should.

I'm not much of an athlete, yet physical activity is very important to me, and to Tim. We go bicycling, hiking in the mountains, camping with the Boy Scouts — activities that I think Becky would enjoy, too, if she were physically capable. As with many achon kids, Becky's weight is a concern, and it would help stave off the possibility of back problems if she were thinner. Like so many other things I saw during my week in Salt Lake, my morning with the DAAA opened my eyes to new possibilities. At home, it seemed that there was just no way of keeping Becky as active as she should be. Here, I began to think that we'd just been looking at it from the wrong angle.

Even inside the bubble of the LPA conference — the one week a year when it's everyone *else* who's different — the average-size world can intrude in unexpected, and not entirely welcome, ways.

At the closing banquet there was a performance by a Native American dance troupe, the same group that performed at the 2002 Olympic ceremonies in Salt Lake City. Following the performance came a certified Awkward Moment, when one of the leaders started talking about the role of little people in Indian folklore as guides to the afterlife. "We very much believe the little people are there to protect us," he said. Another dancer spoke of learning as a child that little people "lived in the forest, they lived in the timber," adding, "We were always taught these stories . . . that if you ever saw these people, you would share very special blessings." He then made "an offering to the little people," presenting a Native American blanket to the outgoing president, Leroy Bankowski, who draped it around his shoulders and smiled gamely.

I probably felt more squeamish about the ceremony than did Bankowski or the little people in the audience. Indeed, a photo of him and the Native American entertainers was later published in *LPA Today*, the organization's newsletter. But there's no getting around, or getting away from, the odd fascination that the outside world has with dwarfs. It's a fascination that can sometimes take a nasty turn — as I learned from Bankowski's successor as LPA president, Matt Roloff, a software developer and sales executive from Helvetia, Oregon.

Unlike most of his predecessors, Roloff was something of a celebrity before his election as president of LPA. He and his wife, Amy Roloff, have overseen the development of a scaled-down theme park on their thirty-four acre farm that has been written up in publications such as the *New York Times*, *People*, and *McCall's*. Matt is also the author of a well-received autobiography, *Against Tall Odds*. He is driven and relentlessly positive, and he and his large family epitomize the image that LPA likes to project about its members. So I was almost surprised (and no, I shouldn't have been) to learn that he, too, has his share of horror stories.

"I literally had someone who was very well-educated — he had thousands of people who worked for him, the vice president of a huge corporation that you've heard of — admit to me after a three-hour plane ride, 'When you first came in, I was petrified. I was going to keep my *Wall Street Journal* open between you and me for as long as possible so I didn't have to engage with you, because I was scared,'" he told me.

I was startled. Surrounding me was the very picture of normality. Matt, forty, and Amy, thirty-nine, were seated across from me. He's diastrophic and gets around with a combination of crutches for short distances and a scooter for longer jaunts. She's achondroplastic. At the next table were their four kids: twins Jeremy and Zachary, twelve; Molly, eight; and Jacob, five. Zach is achon, the rest are average-size.

We were chowing down on McDonald's and Arby's just an hour or so before they would have to make the thirteen-hour drive back to Oregon. But at the moment, they were relaxed. Or as relaxed as the parents of four kids could manage.

Earlier in the week I had attended a talk Amy gave on "Living with Achondroplasia." She was funny, straightforward, dynamic. I learned we had something in common: though she had experienced virtually none of the medical problems that sometimes come with achondroplasia, Zach had had a rough time of it. When he was nine months old he nearly died of RSV, the same respiratory virus that had landed Becky in Massachusetts General Hospital. He didn't need a tracheostomy. But when he was sixteen months old he was diagnosed with hydrocephalus and had to have a shunt surgically inserted in his head. He's had leg-straightening surgery as well. "I have to admit, I was kind of naïve," Amy told us. Indeed, even though she and Matt are both dwarfs — and Matt, as a diastrophic, has had repeated orthopedic surgeries since childhood — they were really not much more prepared for the problems that an achon child could run into than average-size parents would be.

And she said something else, something that showed us just how *on* dwarfs always have to be, how they're never anonymous, can never blend into a crowd, can never sit and brood and shut out the rest of the world. "There are days when I get tired of being at the mall and just don't have the time to be polite and talk to everyone who's curious about my dwarfism," she said. "Yet I know that if I blow them off, they'll form a negative opinion not just about me, but about LPs in general. I still try to be polite. If I'm rude one time, then they'll remember that for life."

I had to remind myself of where I was before I could process what she was saying. We were several days into the conference, and by this point, after being among hundreds of dwarfs, Amy Roloff looked like an absolutely normal, attractive woman. But outside the hotel? Attractive, yes; normal, no.

Whether the attention is negative, as it was on Matt Roloff's flight, or positive, as it is when Amy Roloff is just trying to leave the mall and *make supper*, for crying out loud, it's always there.

If limb-lengthening represents one challenge to group identity, another — and far more common — is what is referred to in LPA circles as a "mixed marriage."

There was a time when a "mixed marriage" might have referred to a couple with two different types of dwarfism, such as Matt and Amy Roloff. Sort of like the old days, when a wedding between, say, an Irish-Catholic and an Italian-Catholic would be referred to as a "mixed marriage." Increasingly, though, the term refers to something considerably more dramatic: a marriage between a short-statured person and an average-size partner.

Such mixed marriages have long been a fact of life, of course, but they were not always accepted within LPA. That appears to have changed. The late Lee Kitchens, a founding father of LPA, told me that at one time he believed it was impossible for a mixed marriage to work out. What changed his mind, he said, were Monica and Neil Pratt. She has SED, is two-foot-eight, and gets around primarily by means of an electric scooter. He is precisely three feet taller than she. When I met them in Salt Lake, he was thirty-five years old; she, thirty-seven. They've been married since 1989.

I had known Monica for several years, mainly by e-mail and an occasional phone call. She's the database coordinator of LPA, keeping track of some twenty-five thousand people who've been in touch with the organization at one time or another, and I depend on her for the information I need to keep LPA Online up to date. The Pratts live in Lubbock, Texas, near the town where Kitchens lived, and who hired her to take over the database when it was beginning to eat up too much of his time.

Monica and Neil met at Angelo State University, her parents' alma mater. Their common interest was religion, and they would spend hours talking about the Bible. But their budding romance almost fell apart before it could begin: she went to Europe the summer after they met, and his letters to her never arrived. When she got back, she avoided him. "He caught me one day and said, 'I want to meet you in the library,'" she told me in her soft, high-pitched voice. "He was, like, really serious, and I thought, 'Oh, my God, he's going to tell me he doesn't want to see me, and why he doesn't want to see me.' So I panicked. But I thought, 'Okay, I can handle this. I'll go.'"

Neil picked up the story. "I asked her if she would consider marrying me, which I guess kind of blew her away. Because we'd never really dated. We'd just been friends and gone to a lot of Bible studies and eaten at the cafeteria together, and had lots of phone conversations."

Monica wanted to take things a little slower, and she warned Neil that a life together would not be as easy as he might imagine. "I said to him, 'You do realize that I have a disability. You do realize that I have dwarfism.' And you know, he's like, 'Yeah, yeah.' But I told him that when I'm in my environment I can function very well. I have my motorized wheelchair. My schedule was set up so I wouldn't have problems. The teachers, the students, were all acclimated to my situation. My dorm room was set up so I could reach stuff. But outside my environment I'm pretty dependent. And also, within the environment of educated people there's not the prejudice and the ignorance. It's not so prevalent. But I step off that campus and it's a whole different world. And that's what I wanted to make sure that he could understand."

I asked Monica whether she had been at all suspicious of Neil's motives. "No," she replied, "because we'd had so many conversations for so long. I had also — I don't know if this is typical or not, but my parents socialized me, big-time. So I was in Brownies, Girl

Scouts, choir, camping, all kinds of activities from age seven. And through that you learn how to gauge people."

But Monica's mother, Eloise Wiegand, admitted that she had her doubts. "I told Neil, 'You just want attention, that's why you want to marry Monica.' I thought that was his motive. And that's that." She paused, then added, "I like Neil. He'll do."

For the past five years Monica and Neil, who's a high-school science teacher, have run workshops at the LPA national conference for people who are in what they call "interspatial relationships." They cover such subjects as how to deal with the dwarf partner's becoming dependent on the average-size partner, how to make a home accessible to both partners, how to introduce the average-size spouse to LPA, and how to introduce the dwarf spouse to average-size family members, friends, and co-workers. "People get over it. There are basic solutions that a lot of people have come to conclusions on," she said.

After studying the LPA database, Monica has concluded that about half of dwarfs who are married have dwarf spouses, and half have average-size spouses. "It's smack in the middle," she said. "But you don't see that at the meetings. Where are they?" The most likely explanation, she continued, is that dwarfs in mixed marriages are far less active in LPA than those who marry other dwarfs.

Thus Monica Pratt has challenged the dwarf community's sense of group identity not just by marrying outside of it, but by insisting on remaining a part of it as well. That LPA has accepted her and Neil so readily says something important about how that sense of identity may be changing. No longer is mixed marriage seen as a threat, as negation, as a running-away from or denial of group identity.

Fourth of July and, as it's been all week, it's mind-alteringly hot in Salt Lake. It's nearly a hundred degrees and as dry as if it were winter and you'd shut yourself in a tiny room with a couple of electric heaters turned up full blast. I'm at Rice-Eccles Stadium, where LPA has scored a block of front-row-center seats for something called the "Red Hot 4th."

The show is a weird combination of schmaltz and patriotism. The first act is a band led by Chuck Negron, the oft-rehabbed former lead singer of Three Dog Night, who rips through a surprisingly energetic and loud set of old hits. He's followed by the alleged headliner, Kenny Loggins, who tries with limited success to rise above his innate flaccidity. We're also treated to three huge military helicopters zooming overhead and an evangelical group of boy singers called Jericho Road. An elderly war hero angrily leads a recitation of the Pledge of Allegiance, the words "under God" spat out in defiance of "some judge in California," as a local news anchorwoman who's emceeing the event puts it.

The show ends with a fireworks display accompanied by the four armed services' official marches. All in all, a far more militaristic display that I ever would have seen back home in liberal Boston.

The image that stays with me, though, is not of the helicopters, not of the flag, and certainly not of Kenny Loggins. Rather, it is of the aisle next to the LPA section, filled with teenage girls, nearly all of them dwarfs, every one of them beautiful and laughing and waving her arms and swaying back and forth to the music. It is a picture of utter normality, a picture that — no matter how smart and happy and popular they may be back home — would be hard to duplicate anywhere but here.

For one week a year they are surrounded by hundreds of people who look like them. In a culture that places outsize importance on appearance, that's important — more important than it should be, but not likely to change anytime soon.

And it's something I'm glad my daughter is part of and can be more a part of as she gets older.

I try to picture Becky in the midst of all this, beautiful not just to us but to others as well. It's a vision that fills me with hope and longing. I find myself wishing she were here, wishing she could meet these girls and exchange e-mail addresses and get all excited about next year's conference.

Becky is heading into what may be the most difficult and painful part of her life — adolescence, when easygoing childhood gives way to the all-consuming need to fit in. Already, her blissful obliviousness is giving way to self-consciousness, to embarrassment over those moments when her difference suddenly becomes blindingly obvious not just to her but to those around her.

When I ask her what she doesn't like about being a dwarf, she is quick to respond that she has to climb on a chair to answer the phone and that she can't go on the older-kid rides at amusement parks. Yet this is superficial, and when Barbara and I press her, she comes up with deeper responses — of how she got rid of the special chair she used to use in school because it singled her out as being different, of how "bad" she feels when younger kids refuse to believe that she's older than they. And when I ask her what she likes about being a dwarf, she really isn't able to come up with anything.

I wish I knew what to tell her. Of course I tell her that there's nothing *wrong* with being a dwarf, that she's just as good and smart and beautiful as anyone else, and that she can be whatever and whoever she wants to be. But this is negation, not affirmation — telling her that her difference isn't a problem, which is not the same as telling her that it's a positive good. And she knows it. What's more, she's smart enough to know that though I'm certainly not lying to her, I *am* gilding the lily.

One day I asked her if she thought she would get married.

"Uh, yeah," she replied. "First I have to find a husband."

When I asked her whether she thought she would marry a "tall" man or a dwarf, she immediately replied that he would be a dwarf.

How come?

"So he's as short as me."

Is that important?

"Uh, yeah. Because tall people don't marry a short person."

Well, sometimes they do.

"A tall person marrying a short person? That doesn't make sense."

Then I asked whether her children would be dwarfs or not.

"Dwarf."

Yeah?

"Because I'm a dwarf. Yeah."

Would that be good?

"Yes."

How come?

"Because when they grow up, they'll be the same size as me."

Now, you're their mother—

"Well, I'm not a mother yet."

I understand. You're their mother, they come to you and they say, "I don't like being a dwarf. I want to be tall." What would you tell them?

"I'd tell them, you can't. You'll never be as tall as a tall person. You'll always be short. And no matter what happens, I'll always love you. How's that?"

That's really good, Becky.

"And lovely?"

Yes.

Shall I leave it there? I could. It's got a nice happily-ever-after ring to it, doesn't it? But there's more.

Do you think that's what they'd want to hear, or do you think they'd be sad to know that they would never grow tall?

"Happy?"

Don't ask me. What do you think?

"I think that they'll be sad."

How come?

"Because they won't be able to reach stuff and I'll have to help them, and they won't be able to go on big rides that they like. So that's why they'll be sad."

So we were back to that. I began to realize that her constant recitation of those two themes was more profound that it seemed — that it spoke to her own unhappiness about being a dwarf, an unhappiness that she already assumes she will pass on to her children. I honestly don't think she dwells on this much; she is essentially a cheerful kid brimming with self-esteem. But there's more to her than that, too, and it's a side of her that I need to recognize and respect. Her heartwarming answer about what she would tell her children was tinged with heartbreak as well.

We all need community. We all need a place of our own. I think we can understand that intellectually, but on that night in Salt Lake City I came to know it in an emotional, visceral way. Becky needs a place where no one — or everyone — needs a stool. Where no one has to stand and watch while their taller friends whoop it up on the big-kid rides. And where they'll see that they can grow up to be parents whose own children's lives will be just as full and happy as those of their average-size peers.

Here, Becky would be just like everyone else. Her dwarfism is just one part of her, and not nearly the most important part. But convincing the world of that will be a lifelong challenge. Every so often she needs to have a chance to relax and be herself and not have to *explain*. To look around and see her own growing sense of self-awareness reflected in the broad, flat faces and short arms and legs of those around her. To understand that she is an individual, but that she is also part of something larger than herself; that she has her own identity and a group identity, and that both are part of who she is. For one week a year, this is where she belongs.

Even if I do worry about those dances.

Acknowledgments

This book has its origins in an e-mail from an extraordinary literary agent, Andrew Blauner. It was May 2001, and the now-defunct magazine *Yahoo! Internet Life* had just published an article about LPA Online, the website of Little People of America, which I have edited since 1998. Andrew took note of my name, tracked me down, and asked if I had ever considered writing a book about dwarfism. For conceiving of *Little People* even before I had, and for tirelessly encouraging me, Andrew has my gratitude and thanks, and then some.

Stephanie Tade, the executive editor of Rodale Books Group, conveyed a sense of excitement that stayed with me throughout the year-long process of research and writing. Chris Potash, who edited the manuscript, pushed me constantly, and passionately, to let Becky's voice be heard and to make the narrative more accessible. Joanna Williams designed the striking cover, and Sarah Lee cleared photo permissions. Sue Ducharme expertly handled the copy-editing.

Since 1991 my professional home has been the *Boston Phoenix*. I value the support that publisher Stephen Mindich and president Barry Morris have given me over the years. *Phoenix* editor Peter

Kadzis deserves special mention for his friendship and enthusiasm for this project.

My friends Susan Ryan-Vollmar, the *Phoenix* news editor, and Ruth Ricker, a past president of Little People of America, read the manuscript and offered valuable suggestions and counsel. Ruth was an important adviser in other ways as well, letting me borrow her collection of books about dwarfism, some of them quite rare, and suggesting people for me to interview.

Betty Adelson, an LPA parent and activist, gave generously of her time, reviewing and helping to correct some of the historical passages.

During the two years that Becky was sick, a troupe of dedicated nurses came into our home and helped take care of her. The ones who stayed with us the longest were Reenee Maloney, Mary Scott Newton, Bernadette Bolling, Lynda Cedrone, June Swartz, and Mary McKenzie. They all have our grateful thanks.

Several years ago a couple with dwarfism whom I had met on the Internet, Fred and Lin Short, of Hartlepool, England, visited us in Danvers. My son, Tim, and I had a terrific time showing them the historical sights of nearby Salem. Fred later sent us a beautiful watercolor of our home that he had painted. Fred and I kept up an e-mail correspondence throughout my research for this book, with him challenging me to get beyond the superficial and confront my deepest feelings.

Tim's sixth-grade Spanish teacher, Hartley Ferguson, put me in touch with Paul and Nancy McNulty, former residents of the Netherlands, who translated a Dutch- and German-language documentary, *Dood Spoor?* ("End of the Line?"), as we watched it in their Danvers home.

Linda Hughes provided me with a videotape of the novelist Armistead Maupin's talk at the 1995 Little People of America national conference in Denver, and of an audiotape of Len Sawisch's presentation at that same conference.

My *Phoenix* colleague Carolyn Clay and her husband, Doug Trees, generously allowed me the use of a spare desk in Doug's architectural office in Hamilton, Massachusetts.

Though parts of this book were researched and written at Doug Trees's office, in our cellar, on our upstairs landing, at Starbucks, in Borders, at Barnes & Noble, and on various road trips, my most comfortable work space was a cubicle with a window view at the Peabody Institute Library in Danvers. I thank the staff for putting up with me.

While putting together the proposal for *Little People*, I read a remarkable book by Michael Bérubé called *Life as We Know It: A Father, a Family, and an Exceptional Child* (Pantheon, 1996), a memoir about raising a son with Down syndrome. Bérubé posits the key question that our culture asks about anyone who is different: "Is this person sufficiently similar to the people we already value?" I hope *Little People* is informed by at least some of the spirit that pervades Bérubé's wise and humane book.

Our children, Timothy and Rebecca, kept me grounded during a year when equilibrium occasionally proved elusive. No father ever had two more perfect kids.

My wonderful wife, Barbara Kennedy, as she has been throughout our twenty-two years of marriage, was my best friend, my lover, my editor and collaborator, and my most sympathetic reader.

Notes

I accessed the websites listed below in 2002 and '03, when I was researching this book. Most of the URLs that are listed are no longer valid.

— DK, 2019

Given the ethics scandals that have plagued journalism in recent years, readers have a right to be skeptical of direct quotations, especially ones produced from memory a considerable time after they were supposedly uttered. For example, in Chapter One I have reproduced several direct quotes from a geneticist with whom we visited a week and a half after Becky's birth. These quotes are reconstructed — that is, I have reproduced them as faithfully as my memory allows but cannot vouch for their complete accuracy. I have tried to keep this practice to a minimum. Nearly all of the direct quotations in this book are from interviews, most of them tape-recorded, a few based on my notes. Quotes from these interviews are verbatim, save for minor changes involving compression and syntax.

Chapter One

Little People of America's definition of dwarfism has been the subject of some debate within the membership, and I have been involved in helping to tweak the language on LPA Online (www.lpaonline.org), the organization's website, which I edited from 1998 until 2005. Under the presidency of Matt Roloff, LPA made it clear that someone with a dwarfism condition who is slightly taller than the four-foot-ten guideline would still be welcomed for membership.

My estimate that there are thirty thousand to fifty thousand people with some type of dwarfism living in the United States is based on an interview I conducted with Angela Muir Van Etten and Robert Van Etten, longtime activists with Little People of America. Several other knowledgeable observers agreed that that was a reasonable figure. The exact number is unknown and, in any case, would depend on the definition of dwarfism that is used.

The statistical definition of dwarfism is an adult height that is in the bottom 0.25 percent of the general population is cited by the medical anthropologist Joan Ablon in *Living with Difference: Families with Dwarf Children* (Praeger, 1988). Ablon's source, in turn, is a 1978 report to the Human Growth Foundation titled *Short Stature: Definition and Estimate of Short Stature in the US Population*, by Thaddeus E. Kelly, Meinhard Robinow, Ann Johanson, Patricia Janku, Fran Kaiser, and W. Shep Fleet.

My estimate of the frequency of achondroplasia — somewhere between one in twenty-six thousand and one in forty thousand births — is taken from a clinical summary published by the Kathryn and Alan C. Greenberg Center for Skeletal Dysplasias, at Johns Hopkins Hospital, on the Web at www.med.jhu.edu /Greenberg.Center/Greenbrg.htm. This estimate has been widely accepted within the dwarf community. The estimates that eighty-five percent of the parents of dwarfs are themselves average-size, and that there are about two hundred different types of dwarfism, are frequently cited by geneticists who specialize in dwarfism. The estimate that two-thirds or more of all cases of dwarfism are caused by achondroplasia is based on conversations with geneticists and people within the dwarf community. Dr. Charles Scott, the former longtime chairman of Little People of America's medical-advisory board, told me that approximately seventy percent of those who attend LPA conferences are achondroplastic. But he cautioned that because achons tend to be healthier and more mobile than people with other types of dwarfism, that figure may not accurately reflect the entire dwarf community.

The roots of the word *achondroplasia* are explained in a March of Dimes fact sheet, available at www.modimes.org.

Chapter Two

The Joan Ablon quote is from her book *Little People in America: The Social Dimensions of Dwarfism* (Praeger, 1984). Ablon later wrote a book on the family dynamics of dwarfism, *Living with Difference* (cited above). Together, the two books represent the most comprehensive attempt to date to describe and explain the dwarf community.

My description of the political-activist branch of the deaf community is based in part on Edward Dolnick's article "Deafness as Culture," which was published in the September 1993 issue of the *Atlantic Monthly.*

Chapter Three

The story of the prehistoric dwarf found wrapped in a woman's — presumably his mother's — arms was reported in the February 1988 edition of *Scientific American* in an article titled "Paleolithic Compassion," by John Horgan; and in the November 9, 1987, issue of the *Washington Post,* in an article headlined "Skeleton of Dwarf Shows Ancients Cared for Disabled," by Boyce Rensberger and Michael Specter. My description of acromesomelic dysplasia is based in part on a conversation with Peggy O'Neill, a three-foot-eight motivational speaker who has the condition and who writes about her life in *Walking Tall: Overcoming Inner Smallness No Matter What Size You Are* (Small Miracles Press, 2002).

Bonnie M. Sampsell's article "Ancient Egyptian Dwarfs" was published in the Fall 2001 edition of *KMT: A Modern Journal of Ancient Egypt.*

The anthropologist Francis E. Johnston's article "Some Observations on the Roles of Achondroplastic Dwarfs through History" was published in the December 1963 edition of the medical journal *Pediatrics.*

Despite its garish style, Hy Roth and Robert Cromie's *The Little People* (Everest House, 1980) contains much valuable information on the history of dwarfs and dwarfism.

The possibility that Richard III was a dwarf is discussed in the August 24, 1991, issue of the *Lancet,* in an unsigned article titled "Richard III: A Royal Pituitary Dwarf?"

The English dwarf Jeffrey Hudson's life story is told in Nick Page's book *Lord Minimus: The Extraordinary Life of Britain's Smallest Man* (St. Martin's Press, 2002).

Norbert Wolf analyzes the place of dwarfs in Velázquez's art in his book *Diego Velázquez, 1599-1600: The Face of Spain* (Taschen, 1999).

The abridged title of the 1863 pamphlet on Charles and Lavinia Stratton's marriage was *Sketch of the Life, Personal Appearance, Character and Manners of Charles S. Stratton, the Man in Miniature, Known as General Tom Thumb, and His Wife, Lavinia Warren Stratton.* That work, along with the autobiographical series that Lavinia Warren wrote for the *New York Tribune Sunday Magazine,* are both online at the Disability History

Museum, www.disabilitymuseum.org.

I am indebted to Robert Bogdan's *Freak Show: Presenting Human Oddities for Amusement and Profit* (University of Chicago Press, 1988) for many of the details regarding the lives of Charles and Lavinia Stratton and P. T. Barnum. Another excellent resource is the documentary film

P. T. Barnum: American Dreamer, part of the A&E "Biography" series, which I saw during my visit to the Barnum Museum, in Bridgeport, Connecticut. I also consulted Mertie E. Romaine's *General Tom Thumb and His Lady* (William S. Sullwold Publishing, 1976).

Chapter Four

The website that I describe concerning Alexander Katan is based in Brazil, and the text is in Portuguese. The address is www.internau.psi.br/pp/mauthausen /pseudo. htm. I was able to obtain an imperfect but useful translation through Google. I have subsequently found much of the same information at other locations on the Web.

The horrors of the Mauthausen concentration camp are described on the websites of the Austrian government's Mauthausen Memorial (www.mauthausen-memorial .at); the KZ Mauthausen-Gusen Info-Pages (www.gusen.org); and the "Forgotten Camps" project of a Jewish genealogical site called JewishGen.org (www.jewishgen .org/Forgotten Camps/Camps/MauthausenEng.html).

The story of William Henry "Zip" Johnson has been recounted by a number of historians. I consulted Bogdan's *Freak Show* and A. H. Saxon's *P. T. Barnum: The Legend and the Man* (Columbia University Press, 1989).

The lives of Sir Francis Galton and Gregor Mendel are discussed in "Building Superman," by David Reich, in the February 10, 2002, issue of the *New York Times Book Review* (Reich reviewed Nicholas Wright Gillham's biography *A Life of Sir Francis Galton*); and in Simon Mawer's novel *Mendel's Dwarf* (Harmony Books, 1998).

Rosemarie Garland Thomson's essay "Seeing the Disabled: Visual Rhetorics of Disability in Popular Photography" was published in *The New Disability History: American Perspectives*, edited by Paul K. Longmore and Lauri Umansky (New York University Press, 2001).

I have not seen the movie *The Black Stork*, but both it and its bizarre impresario, Dr. Harry Haiselden, are described in *The Disability Rights Movement: From Charity to Confrontation*, by Doris Zames Fleischer and Frieda Zames (Temple University Press, 2001); and in *Beyond Affliction: The Disability History Project*, a 1998 public-radio documentary series produced by Laurie Block (founder of the online Disability History Museum), Jay Allison, and John Crowley. Both of those works, in turn, cite Martin S. Pernick's *The Black Stork: Eugenics and the Death of "Defective" Babies in American Medicine and Motion Pictures Since 1915* (Oxford University Press, 1996).

Carrie Bruck's plight — and Justice Holmes's heartless reaction to it — are described in Joseph P. Shapiro's *No Pity: People with Disabilities Forging a New Civil Rights Movement* (Times Books, 1993).

I relied primarily on three sources for my description of the Nazis' sterilization and "euthanasia" programs: Robert Jay Lifton's *The Nazi Doctors: Medical Killing and the Psychology of Genocide* (Basic Books, 1986); Hugh Gregory Gallagher's *By Trust Betrayed: Patients, Physicians, and the License to Kill in the Third Reich* (Holt, 1990); and *The Mentally and Physically Handicapped: Victims of the Nazi Era*, a publication of the United States Holocaust Memorial Museum.

Perla Ovitz, the central figure in the documentary *Liebe Perla*, was interviewed by Yehuda Koren for the *Telegraph Magazine*, which is based in Britain. That article was later reprinted in the November 1999 issue of *Hadassah Magazine.*

Gerald L. Posner and John Ware are the authors of *Mengele: The Complete Story* (McGraw-Hill, 1986).

Sara Nomberg-Przytyk is the author of *Auschwitz: True Tales from a Grotesque Land* (University of North Carolina Press, 1985).

Ursula Hegi is the author of *Stones from the River* (Scribner, 1994).

Chapter Five

The Reverend Martin Marty's thoughts on Jesus and the disabled are included in an interview he did for a book called *How I Pray: People of Different Religions Share with Us That Most Sacred and Intimate Act of Faith*, edited by Jim Castelli (Ballantine, 1994).

I found the Reverend John Yates's sermon on Jesus and the disabled on the website of his church, the Falls Church, at www.thefallschurch.org/SERMONS /1999sermons/990228jy.htm.

Hugh Gregory Gallagher writes about Jesus and the disabled in *By Trust Betrayed* (cited above).

I had heard that the word *handicap* was derived from *cap in hand*, and that struck me as both logical and a characteristically degrading way of thinking about the disabled. But when I started to research the etymology, I found an entry on the well-respected urban-legends website Snopes.com debunking that interpretation. (See www.snopes.com/language/offense/handicap.htm.) In addition, the *American Heritage Dictionary* (fourth edition, 2000) says that *handicap* is "[f]rom obsolete *hand in cap*, a game in which forfeits were held in a cap."

Peter Hall's and Laurie Block's comments are taken from the radio documentary *Beyond Affliction.*

The stories by the Bosnian refugees were told in an article by Stephen Kinzer headlined "Terrorized Human Tide Overwhelms Relief Camp," which appeared on July 15, 1995, in the *New York Times.*

Although the Reverend Paul Stevens Lynn's comments are from a telephone interview I conducted with him, I first learned about him in an article by the Reverend Alton M. Motter in the May-September 1999 issue of *LPA Today*, the newsletter of Little People of America.

Rabbi Harold Kushner's *When Bad Things Happen to Good People* has been a phenomenon since it was first published in 1981. The twentieth-anniversary edition, issued in 2001, was published by Schocken Books.

The passage by the Reverend Forrest Church is from "Open Up to the Mystery," published in the September-October 2000 issue of the *UU World*, the magazine of the Unitarian Universalist Association. I was also helped by Church's book *Life Lines: Holding on (and Letting Go)* (Beacon Press, 1996), in which he offers this wonderful explanation of the difference between his (and my) thinking and that of atheists: "Unlike them, I believe in what I cannot know, the God beyond God, not omnipotent and omniscient — these are human constructs — but ineffable and inscrutable, subject neither to human description nor human understanding. When I say I believe in God, God is not God's name. God is our name for that which is greater than all and yet present in each, a mystery that cannot be named or known." He adds: "None of this makes sense. I know that."

The origins of the Kaleigh Mulligan program are described in a *Boston Globe* article headlined "Law Aids Families with Disabled Children," by Anne Wyman, published on December 21, 1989.

Chapter Six

Erving Goffman lays out his analysis of stigmatized groups and individuals in *Stigma: Notes on the Management of Spoiled Identity* (Simon & Schuster, 1963).

My discussion of the history of the disability-rights movement is informed by several excellent studies. Particularly valuable is Joseph P. Shapiro's *No Pity* (cited on page 285). My estimate of nearly 50 million disabled Americans is based on Shapiro, who, writing a decade earlier, placed the number somewhere between 35 million and 43 million.

Although I interviewed Paul Steven Miller, I relied on Shapiro's *No Pity* in describing Miller's representation of television anchor Bree Walker Lampley. My other secondary sources on disability rights are Doris Zames Fleischer and Frieda Zames's *The Disability Rights Movement*, especially for their account of the League of the Physically Handicapped; and the radio documentary *Beyond Affliction*. The remarks by President George H. W. Bush at the signing ceremony for the Americans with Disabilities Act are taken from a *Washington Post* account of July 27, 1990, headlined "In Emotion-Filled Ceremony, Bush Signs Rights Law for America's Disabled," by Ann Devroy.

The story of dwarf employees who helped build B-24 bombers for Ford is told in "Little People with Big Jobs," by Dave Elsila, published in the October 1997 issue of the United Auto Workers' *Solidarity* magazine.

The early history of Little People of America is recounted in the organization's twenty-fifth-anniversary souvenir book, published in 1982 and distributed to members at that year's national conference in Reno, Nevada — the site of the first gathering of Billy Barty's fledgling Midgets of America in 1957. Barty served as the writer and executive editor of the book.

Chapter Seven

Parts of Barnum's 1855 autobiography, *The Life of P. T. Barnum: Written by Himself*, are online at the Disability History Museum, www.disabilitymuseum .org. If you search for the word *midget*, you will find nothing; but if you search for *dwarf* you will find several references to Charles Stratton. This is of particular significance because Stratton, who as a growth-hormone-deficient dwarf had the same proportions as an average-size person, fits the classic definition of *midget*. This clearly shows that the M-word was not in use at that time.

Robert Bogdan discusses the words *dwarf* and *midget* in the context of circus and sideshow performers in his book *Freak Show*.

Angela Muir Van Etten's autobiography is *Dwarfs Don't Live in Doll Houses* (Adaptive Living, 1988).

Chapter Eight

Dr. Steven Kopits was profiled in a cover story in the *Washington Post Magazine* on December 9, 1984, titled "Dr. Steven Kopits: The Little People's God," by Brad Lemley, with photographs by Margaret Thomas. Kopits was a devout Catholic, and the title was a source of some irritation to him, according to his brother, George Kopits, who eulogized him on June 22, 2002. "He resented the well-meaning label on the cover of the *Washington Post* characterizing him as the 'God of the Little People,'" George Kopits said. "Steven knew well the difference between God and surgeons . . . Indeed, he often declared that he was acting merely as an instrument of Divine Providence." George Kopits's eulogy can be found at the website of the Little People's Research Fund, an organization begun by Steven Kopits, at www.lprf.org.

In addition to interviewing Dr. Michael Ain and observing him as he worked on two separate occasions, I also consulted two media profiles: "Aiming High," by Melissa Hendricks, with photographs by Mike Ciesielski, published by *Johns Hopkins Magazine* in April 1999; and "The Doctor Who Almost Wasn't," broadcast by the ABC News show *20/20* on November 19, 1999, reported by Dr. Tim Johnson and produced by Callie Crossley.

Joan Hawkins's essay "'One of Us': Tod Browning's *Freaks*" is included in *Freakery: Cultural Spectacles of the Extraordinary Body*, edited by Rosemarie Garland Thomson (New York University Press, 1996).

I found three pieces helpful to my understanding of *De eso no se habla* ("I Don't Want to Talk About It"): an untitled review by Karen Jaehne in the Winter 1994 issue of *Film Quarterly*; a profile of the director, Maria Luisa Bemberg, headlined "Political Subtext in a Fairy Tale from a Feminist," by Peter Brunette, published in the *New York Times* on September 25, 1994; and a review of the film, headlined "Recognizing People Who Have the Courage to Be Different," by Janet Maslin, published in the *New York Times* on September 30, 1994.

Chapter Nine

The *People* magazine story on Gillian Mueller, "Long on Courage," by Kim Hubbard and Giovanna Breu, with photographs by Mimi Cotter, was published on February 17, 1992. Mueller and her limb-lengthening surgery have been written about on many occasions over the years. As I am something of a connoisseur of media excess, I have to say that my favorite headline, which Mueller showed me in a scrapbook in Dr. Dror Paley's office, is "Tragic Gillian," from the *Globe*, a supermarket tabloid.

Ralph Keyes wrote about discrimination against short people in *The Height of Your Life* (Little Brown, 1980). I also consulted Leslie F. Martel and Henry B. Biller's *Stature and Stigma: The Biopsychological Development of Short Males* (Lexington Books, 1987).

The study of self-esteem and quality of life is titled *Living with Achondroplasia in an Average-Sized World: An Assessment of Quality of Life*, by Sarah E. Gollust, Richard E. Thompson, Holly C. Gooding, and Barbara B. Biesecker.

The study of how achondroplastic adults perceive their physical and mental health is titled "Functional Health Status of Adults with Achondroplasia," by Nizar N. Mahomed, Mark Spellmann, and Michael J. Goldberg. It was published in the June 16, 1998, issue of the *American Journal of Medical Genetics* (volume 78, issue 1).

One of the best lay explanations of limb-lengthening is included in an article titled "Up with People," by David Berreby, published by *The New Republic* on April 29, 1996. Other articles I found tended to be too technical, too old to be reliable, or both. However, the methods used by Dr. Dror Paley and Dr. John Herzenberg at their International Center for Limb Lengthening, in Baltimore, are explained in great detail on their website, www.limblengthening.org.

The Little People of America medical-advisory board's statement on limb-lengthening, Gillian Mueller's essay, and other resources on the procedure can be found in the LPA Online Library at www.lpaonline.org/resources_library.html.

Chapter Ten

There are many books on ADHD, most of which either passionately advocate the use of medication or are aflame with dire warnings against its use. By contrast, Dr. Lawrence H. Diller's *Running on Ritalin: A Physician Reflects on Children, Society, and Performance in a Pill* (Bantam Books, 1998) takes a restrained, balanced approach. I also first learned about central-auditory-processing disorder in *Running on Ritalin.*

When the Brain Can't Hear: Unraveling the Mystery of Auditory Processing Disorders, by Teri James Bellis (Pocket Books, 2002), is a good guide to this subject. Also helpful is "Central Auditory Processing Disorder: When Is Evaluation Referral Indicated?" by Sandra Cleveland, the Northeastern University audiologist who was in charge of Becky's evaluation. That article was published in the October 1997 issue of *The ADHD Report.* It is also available online at www.ldonline.org/ld_ indepth/process_deficit/adhdreport_capd.html.

Chapter Eleven

A profile of Anthony Soares was published by the Columbia News Service, a student news agency sponsored by the Columbia University Graduate School of Journalism, on February 22, 2002. The piece, titled "Politician Puts His Mind to Bigger Issues," by Brett Tomlinson, is online at www.jrn.columbia.edu /studentwork/cns/2002-02-14/57.asp.

The controversy over Steve Vento, a dwarf who worked in a Mexican restaurant by serving chips and salsa from a sombrero on top of his head, was written about by Chris Lydgate in the weekly newspaper *Willamette Week*. Lydgate's article, headlined "Dwarf vs. Dwarf: The Little People of America Want Respect and They're Fighting Each Other to Get It," was published on June 30, 1999, on the eve of LPA's annual conference, which was held that year in nearby Portland, Oregon.

Armistead Maupin's novel *Maybe the Moon* was published by Harper-Collins in 1992. He spoke of his relationship with the late Tamara De Treaux in an interview with London's *Sunday Mail.* The article, titled "*E.T.* Dwarf Finds Fame . . . at Last," was written by Janice Turner, and was published on February 28, 1993. Maupin also discussed his friendship with De Treaux at the LPA national conference in Denver in 1995. I was able to view a videotape of his talk.

Chapter Twelve

The discovery of the genetic mutation that causes achondroplasia was announced in the scientific journal *Cell* on July 29, 1994. The article, titled "Mutations in the Transmembrane Domain of FGFR3 Cause the Most Common Genetic Form of Dwarfism, Achondroplasia," was written by Rita Shiang, Leslie M. Thompson, Ya-Zhen Zhu, Deanna M. Church, Thomas J. Fielder, Maureen Bocian, Sara T. Winokur, and John J. Wasmuth. It is, as you might imagine, completely impenetrable to the lay reader, including this one.

A November 5, 1994, article in *Science News* titled "Beyond the Genome: The Ethics of DNA Testing," by Kathy A. Fackelmann, discusses several ethical dilemmas regarding prenatal screening, including a hypothetical achondroplastic couple who had informed their doctor that they would choose abortion if they learned their child would not be a dwarf. In April 2000, the *Journal of Medical Ethics*, in an article titled "Disability, Gene Therapy, and Eugenics — a Challenge to John Harris," by Solveig Magnus Reindal, discussed another hypothetical achondroplastic couple, this one wishing to implant an achondroplastic embryo via in vitro fertilization. "Is it defensible," Reindal asks, "for a doctor to override the wishes of the couple and implant the embryos without achondroplasia rather than those with achondroplasia?" To which the obvious answer would seem to be: "Of course not."

The study showing that two percent of achondroplastic couples would consider abortion if they learned their child would not be a dwarf is titled "Issues Surrounding Prenatal Testing for Achondroplasia," by Holly C. Gooding, Karina Boehm, Richard Thompson, Don Hadley, Clair Francomano, and Barbara Bowles Biesecker. I have not seen their unpublished manuscript, but their findings were reported in an article titled "Unintended Messages: The Ethics of Teaching Genetic Dilemmas," by Holly Gooding, Benjamin Wilfond, Karina Boehm, and Barbara Bowles Biesecker, which was published in the March-April 2002 issue of the *Hastings Center Report.*

Adrienne Asch discusses her views on selective abortion in *Prenatal Testing and Disability Rights*, edited by Erik Parens and Asch (Georgetown University Press, 2000). I draw from the introductory essay, which she wrote with Parens, titled "The Disability Rights Critique of Prenatal Genetic Testing: Reflections and Recommendations," and from an essay she wrote by herself titled "Why I Haven't Changed My Mind about Prenatal Diagnosis: Reflections and Refinements."

Peter Singer's views on infanticide are laid out in astoundingly graphic detail in *Should the Baby Live? The Problem of Handicapped Infants* (Oxford University Press,

1985), which he co-wrote with Helga Kuhse. At one point they write, "Quite often a defect which would have warranted abortion during pregnancy is not discovered until birth. Has the situation then changed so critically that it is now horrific to contemplate ending a life which three months previously could have been ended with little controversy?" I think most normal people would say, "Well, uh, yes."

Michael Specter's understated but devastating profile of Singer, "The Dangerous Philosopher," appeared in the *New Yorker* on September 6, 1999.

Dorothy C. Wertz presented the findings of her study on attitudes toward disability in an essay titled "Drawing Lines: Notes for Policymakers," which was published in the book *Prenatal Testing and Disability Rights*, cited above.

Little People of America's views on genetic testing are spelled out in "Do We Really Want This? Little People of America Inc. Comes to Terms with Genetic Testing," by Ruth E. Ricker (1995), and in an article titled "Little People of America: Position Statement on Genetic Discoveries in Dwarfism" (1996). Both are available in the LPA Online Library, at www.lpaonline.org/resources_library .html.

Gregory Stock's book *Redesigning Humans* was published by Houghton Mifflin in 2002.

Clair Francomano wrote about the genetics of achondroplasia in "Clinical Implications of Basic Research: The Genetic Basis of Dwarfism," published in the *New England Journal of Medicine* on January 5, 1995.

An excellent introduction to the science of genetics is Matt Ridley's *Genome: The Autobiography of a Species in 23 Chapters* (Perennial, 2000).

The link between cadaver-derived human growth hormone, or hGH, and Creutzfeldt-Jakob disease has been widely reported. I relied on an article by David Davis, titled "Cut Short," that appeared on the website of *Mother Jones* magazine on March 23, 2000. The article can be found at www.motherjones.com /news_wire /short.html.

The possible link between hGH and cancer was reported by NBC News correspondent Robert Bazell on July 25, 2002, and by the BBC on July 26, 2002 (news.bbc.co .uk/1/hi/health/2150953.stm).

Simon Mawer's novel *Mendel's Dwarf* is the story of Benedict Lambert, a geneticist with achondroplasia who is a descendant of the pioneering geneticist Gregor

Mendel. Mawer offers an extensive discussion of the history of the eugenics movement and the discovery of the mutation that causes achondroplasia that is entirely accurate except for one large fictional conceit: he attributes the discovery to Lambert rather than to John Wasmuth and his colleagues. *Mendel's Dwarf* is not only a remarkable piece of fiction, but it helped inform my views on eugenics and science as well.

Chapter Thirteen

Kurt Vonnegut's novel *Cat's Cradle* was originally published in 1963 by Holt, Rinehart & Winston.

John Wolin wrote about his first Little People of America conference in an article titled "Dwarf Like Me," which was published in *Tropic* magazine, part of the *Miami Herald*, on January 24, 1993.

Although I did not attend LPA's 1995 national conference, I was able to listen to an audiotape of Len Sawisch's presentation.

Cara Egan's master's thesis is titled *LPA, Inc.: Coming of Age in the Policy Arena.* She researched it and wrote it while a student at the School of Hygiene and Public Health at Johns Hopkins University. Egan also wrote a "My Turn" essay for *Newsweek* titled "The Seven Dwarfs and I," published on September 9, 1991. It was one of the first pieces on dwarfism that Barbara and I ever read following Becky's being diagnosed with achondroplasia.

Matt Roloff's autobiography, co-written with Tracy Sumner, is *Against Tall Odds: Being a David in a Goliath World* (Multnomah Publishers, 1999). He maintains his own website, which contains a considerable amount of information about his farm and theme park, at www.mattroloff.com.

About the Author

Dan Kennedy is a professor of journalism at Northeastern University in Boston and is a nationally known commentator on media issues. He is the author of three books on the future of journalism, the most recent of which, *What Works in Community News: Media Startups, News Deserts, and the Future of the Fourth Estate* (with Ellen Clegg), will be published in 2024. His blog, *Media Nation*, is online at dankennedy.net.

From 1994 until 2005, Kennedy was the media columnist for *The Boston Phoenix*. Prior to that he worked as a staff reporter and editor for *The Daily Times Chronicle* of Woburn, Massachusetts. In 2019 he received the Yankee Quill Award from the New England Academy of Journalists in recognition of his contributions to the profession, and in 2018 he received the James W. Carey Award for Outstanding Journalism from the Media Ecology Association. Previously he received the National Press Club's Arthur Rowse Award for Press Criticism (2001) and the media-reporting award from the Association of Alternative Newsweeklies (1999).

Kennedy was born and grew up in Middleborough, Massachusetts. He and his wife, Barbara Kennedy, live in West Medford, Massachusetts. They are the parents of two adult children.

Made in the USA
Monee, IL
11 November 2026

68342112R00163